Miscommunicating the COVID-19 Pandemic

This book tackles the infodemic—the rapid, widespread diffusion of false, misleading, or inaccurate information about the disease and its ramifications—triggered by the COVID-19 pandemic. With a focus on four Asian societies, the book compares and analyzes the spread of COVID-19 misinformation and its broad impacts on the public in Beijing, Hong Kong, Taipei, and Singapore.

Providing both a comprehensive overview of the phenomenon of misinformation and cross-societal analyses of patterns, the book features in-depth analyses of the prevalence of COVID-19 misinformation and engagement and explores its consequences in an Asian context. The book sheds light on these key questions:

- What types of infodemic messages circulate widely on popular social media platforms?
- What factors account for exposure to and engagement with debunked yet popular COVID-19 misinformation?
- How does exposure to widely circulated COVID-19 misinformation affect people's beliefs, attitudes, and adoption of preventive measures to cope with the pandemic?
- How do macro social differences condition the diffusion and impacts of COVID-19 misinformation?
- What intervention strategies can counter the misinformation?

Presenting scientific insights and empirical findings on the pressing issues about infodemic, this book will be of great interest to students and researchers of communication studies, political science, public health, crisis communication, and Asian Studies, as well as policymakers and practitioners who wish to acquire cutting-edge, evidence-based knowledge about combating misinformation during a global pandemic.

Ran Wei is Chair Professor in the School of Communication of Hong Kong Baptist University, a retired Professor of the Chinese University of Hong Kong, and a Distinguished Professor Emeritus of the University of South Carolina, USA.

Routledge Advances in Internationalizing Media Studies
Edited by Daya Thussu
Hong Kong Baptist University

Miscommunicating the COVID-19 Pandemic

An Asian Perspective

Ran Wei with Ven-Hwei Lo, Yi-Hui
Christine Huang, Dong Dong, Hai Liang,
Guanxiong Huang, and Sibo Wang

Routledge
Taylor & Francis Group

LONDON AND NEW YORK

First published 2024
by Routledge
4 Park Square, Milton Park, Abingdon, Oxon OX14 4RN

and by Routledge
605 Third Avenue, New York, NY 10158

Routledge is an imprint of the Taylor & Francis Group, an informa business

© 2024 Ran Wei

British Library Cataloguing-in-Publication Data
A catalogue record for this book is available from the British Library

Library of Congress Cataloging-in-Publication Data
Names: Wei, Ran, 1962– author.
Title: Miscommunicating the COVID-19 pandemic : an Asian perspective /
by Ran Wei with Ven-Hwei Lo, Yi-Hui Christine Huang, Dong Dong,
Hai Liang, Guanxiong Huang, Sibo Wang
Description: New York : Routledge, 2024. |
Series: Routledge advances in internationalizing media studies | Includes
bibliographical references and index. |
Identifiers: LCCN 2023015605 (print) | LCCN 2023015606 (ebook) |
ISBN 9781032408880 (hardback) | ISBN 9781032410470 (paperback) |
ISBN 9781003355984 (ebook)
Subjects: LCSH: COVID-19 Pandemic, 2020—-Political aspects—Asia. |
COVID-19 Pandemic, 2020—Social aspects—Asia. | COVID-19 Pandemic,
2020– , in mass media. | Misinformation—Asia.
Classification: LCC RA644.C67 W44 2023 (print) | LCC RA644.C67
(ebook) | DDC 362.1962/41440095—dc23/eng/20230607
LC record available at https://lccn.loc.gov/2023015605
LC ebook record available at https://lccn.loc.gov/2023015606

ISBN: 978-1-032-40888-0 (hbk)
ISBN: 978-1-032-41047-0 (pbk)
ISBN: 978-1-003-35598-4 (ebk)

DOI: 10.4324/9781003355984

Typeset in Sabon LT Pro
by codeMantra

Contents

Contributors

Ran Wei (PhD), an internationally acclaimed scholar in communications research, is a Chair Professor in the School of Communication of Hong Kong Baptist University, Hong Kong, a retired Professor of the Chinese University of Hong Kong, and a Distinguished Professor Emeritus of the University of South Carolina, USA. His research focuses on media psychology and effects, cognitive bias and perception, and mobile communication. His refereed publications include nine books, 23 book chapters, and 90+ peer-reviewed articles in top-tier journals such as *Communication Research*, *Journal of Computer Mediated Communication, New Media & Society*, and *Media Psychology*. Stanford's John Ioannidis' team ranked him as one of the world's top 2% scientists; Elsevier, as "Most Cited Chinese Scholars in Social Sciences"; and the Canadian Council of Academies as among the top 5% most cited scholars in communication. He was inducted as an ICA Fellow in May 2022. He has served as Editor-in-Chief of *Journal of Information Society* and *Mass Communication & Society*, is currently Editor of *Communication and Society* (an ICA-affiliated journal), a founding board member of *Mobile Media and Communication*, and a member of 12 editorial boards of leading journals in the field. He was chair of *Communication and Technology*, ICA's largest division from 2020 to 2022, and was President of the *Chinese Communication Association* (an ICA affiliate).

Chapter Lead Authors

Dong Dong (PhD) is an Assistant Professor in the Jockey Club School of Public Health and Primary Care at the Chinese University of Hong Kong. Her research interests include health communication, science and technology studies, health equity, and social justice.

Guanxiong Huang (PhD) is an Associate Professor in the Department of Media and Communication at the City University of Hong Kong. Her research interests include health communication, media psychology, and persuasive technologies.

Yi-Hui Christine Huang (PhD) is a Chair Professor in the Department of Media and Communication and the Associate Dean of College of Liberal Arts and Social Sciences at the City University of Hong Kong. Her research interests include strategic communication and risk communication.

Hai Liang (PhD) is an Associate Professor in the School of Journalism and Communication at the Chinese University of Hong Kong. His research interests include computational social science, political communication, and public health.

Ven-Hwei Lo (PhD) is a Visiting Professor in the Department of Journalism at the Hong Kong Baptist University. His research expertise falls into two streams: effects of mass media and journalism studies.

Sibo Wang (PhD) is an Assistant Professor in the Department of Systems Engineering and Engineering Management at the Chinese University of Hong Kong. His research focuses on database and data mining.

Contributing Co-authors

Anfan Chen (PhD) is a Postdoctoral Fellow in the School of Journalism and Communication, The Chinese University of Hong Kong, and an Associate Professor in the Department of Science Communication, University of Science and Technology of China. His research interests include computational communication, science communication, and political communication.

Jing Guo (MA) is a PhD candidate in the School of Journalism and Communication, the Chinese University of Hong Kong. Her research interests include political communication and health communication with a focus on social media.

Jun Li (PhD) is a Postdoctoral Fellow in the Department of Journalism at Hong Kong Baptist University. Her research interests focus on public administration and political communication.

Miao Lu (PhD) is an Assistant Professor in the Department of Cultural Studies, Lingnan University. Her research interests include digital cultures and global China studies.

Sai Wang (PhD) is a Research Assistant Professor in the Department of Interactive Media at Hong Kong Baptist University. Her research interests include computer-mediated communication, media psychology, and human-computer interaction.

Wenting Yu (PhD) is a Research Assistant Professor in the Department of Journalism at Hong Kong Baptist University. Her research interests include computer-mediated communication, public opinion, and health communication.

Yan Zeng (MA) is a Research Assistant at the Jockey Club School of Public Health and Primary Care at the Chinese University of Hong Kong. Her research interests include the sociology of health and illness, and the quality of life of patients with rare diseases.

Grace Xiao Zhang (PhD) is an Assistant Professor in the Department of Journalism and Communication, Hong Kong Shue Yan University. Her research interests include social media studies, media effects, marketing communication, and health communication.

Acknowledgments

The completion of this collaborative book from conception to printing truly reflects teamwork. The eight-member team that I assembled for a funded CRF (Collaborative Research Fund) project about diffusion and impacts of the infodemic in Spring 2020 has expanded considerably with the addition of several new members over the course of completing this book. Six co-PIs are lead authors, assisted by post-doc or graduate students who contributed a chapter or two. I thank them for their contributions and for bearing with my nagging and constant reminders of due dates. Without teamwork, there would be no book.

Collaboration among scholars is highly touted, but in practice, interdisciplinary collaboration cutting across different fields is rare for a number of reasons. I'm fortunate to know and work with every member of this CRF project team. My co-PIs are brilliant scholars in their own research; having them on the team has enabled me to accomplish something of greater significance than I could achieve alone. Each chapter showcases the academic excellence of the contributors. I have learned from each member of the team during our three-year collaboration. Together, I believe we have made a contribution to the field and society with this book devoted to studying misinformation about COVID-19 on social media.

The data presented in this book was based primarily on large-scale fieldwork, including big data scaped from Weibo, web survey data of 4,094 respondents in Beijing, Hong Kong, Singapore, and Taipei, data from telephone surveys of another 4,114 respondents, and the 80 participants of 16 focus groups in four of Asia's leading cities. The use of different research methods has allowed us to cross-validate the results and integrate the key findings with a cross-societal perspective. As far as I know, the scale and scope of such work are unprecedented in the Asian region.

The book is structured into three sections: FDI (Foundation, Diffusion, and Impacts). In the first section, Chapter 1 provides the conceptual foundation with an overview of the research design. In the second section, Chapters 2–5 trace the emergence of misinformation related to COVID-19 and examine its diffusion patterns through exposure and sharing on social media platforms in the four cities. The third section—Chapters 6–11—examines the public harms of widely diffused misinformation. The coauthors investigated a range of adverse effects of encountering COVID-19 misinformation on citizens' emotions, cognition, attitudes, and behavior. Each chapter ends with evidence-based insights and recommendations for policy actions. An Asian perspective that emerges from the key findings is discussed in the concluding chapter—Chapter 12.

The work we put into completing this book is cumulative. As survey data and focus group discussion transcripts became available at different stages of our fieldwork, we drafted a few stand-alone papers to make full use of the fresh data. In the process, my team and I presented and published four papers for international and regional conferences. Based on themes and topical relevance, these papers were incorporated into the book. Specifically, we cited Wei et al. (2022) in Chapters 1 and 8. Trust in government in Chapter 7 was informed by a paper prepared for the ICA conference (see Huang et al., 2023). Chapters 6 and 10 included elements from a stand-alone paper presented at the ICA 2022 conference in Paris (i.e., Lo et al., 2022). Another ICA paper (Wei et al., 2023) focusing on information overload during the pandemic was partially incorporated into Chapter 9.

Completing a book manuscript is huge commitment, including sacrificing coffee hours with friends, long weekends, and lost time with families. I wish to give my thanks to the families and friends of the authors and co-authors who are not listed here, but their support has been crucial to the completion of this book in 12 months. Mr. Bruce Burton, the copyeditor and long-time friend of ours, is another person whose name does not show. His critical reading and provocative comments have made the entire manuscript more readable and insightful.

Last, but not least, I would like to thank Ms. Susanne Richardson of Routledge. The idea and spark for this book came from an intensive email exchange with her during the 2021 ICA conference. I'm grateful for her enthusiastic support and her professionalism in handling the publishing of this book project.

Ran Wei

The work described in this book was supported by a grant from the Research Grants Council of the Hong Kong Special Administrative Region, China (Project No. C4158-20G).

References

Huang, Y., Wei, R., Lo, V., Sun, J., Cai, Q., & Yu, W. (2023, May 24–29). *COVID messaging in context: The role of information environment in understanding vaccination hesitancy in four Asian cities* [Paper presentation]. 73rd Annual ICA Conference, Toronto, Canada.

Lo, V., Wei, R., Lu, M., Grace, Z., & Qiu, J. (2022, May 26–30). *A comparative study of the impact of digital media environments, information processing, and presumed influence on behavioral responses to COVID-19 misinformation in four Asian cities* [Paper presentation]. 72nd Annual ICA Conference, Paris, France.

Wei, R., Guo, J., Wang, S., & Huang, Y. (2022). The role of digital information accessibility in shaping the relationships of exposure to COVID-19 misinformation and cognitive and attitudinal effects in Asia. *Communication & Society*, 62, 127–159. http://www.cschinese.com/issueArticle.asp?P_No=93&CA_ID=708

Wei, R., Lo, V., Guo, J. & Yu, W. (2023, May 24–29). *An unhelpful chain: From information overload to vaccine mistrust under different national anti-COVID strategies* [Paper presentation]. 73rd Annual ICA Conference, Toronto, Canada.

1   Introduction

Ran Wei

Infodemic and the Global Public Health Crisis

Seemingly true but false information about COVID-19 is everywhere on leading social media platforms; it has appeared in all sizes, shapes, and colors (e.g., rumors, hoaxes, fake news). Over the past three years, we have endured a global pandemic that has spread to more than 200 countries. We have also lived with a tsunami of misinformation. Rumors concerning China, where COVID-19 first appeared, surged on social media, especially in the early stage of the outbreak in Wuhan, such as SARS-CoV-2 is a lab-edited and leaked from the laboratory (Chen et al., 2020). In the United Kingdom, some 77 cellular towers were set on fire by believers of the claim that ultrafast wireless technology "5G causes the coronavirus" (Hamilton, 2020).

Half-truths about COVID are not just annoying; consuming such factually incorrect and misleading information has real consequences. Here are a number of real-life stories:

- *Misguided Recommendations.* In Hong Kong, a health expert posted a recommendation to concerned residents: Arm yourself with a high-power hair dryer to blow away the corona virus. The post went viral, causing a good deal of confusion among the public. Residents in Beijing panicked after viewing a widely circulated video which claimed residuals on facial masks could cause cancer if the masks weren't shaken before putting them on. After viewing a post on social media during the early stage of the COVID-19 outbreak, Singapore residents reported increased rinsing of their noses with saline solutions (Kim & Tandoc, 2022).
- *False Cures.* In Singapore, a post circulated on Facebook touted a controversial medicine called "ivermectin" to prevent or treat COVID-19 infections. A local church pastor informed the news media that the mother of a church goer was hospitalized after taking ivermectin. A pop singer in Taiwan was arrested for reposting on Instagram that "Weed Kills Corona Virus." He said that he believed the post he saw on an American friend's page because it looked like a real screenshot of breaking news on TV.

DOI: 10.4324/9781003355984-1

- *Vaccine Hesitancy*. The vaccination rate was low among elderly Taiwanese and Hong Kongers because they were concerned about side effects. During that time, a tweet by Dr. Robert Malone, a co-inventor of mRNA, gained popularity on PTT (a popular social media site). The tweet said Malone was outraged by the FDA's approval of the vaccine without full consideration of its side effects. In a podcast on YouTube that went viral globally, he expressed regret for taking the shot. Meanwhile, China's Weibo circulated an unverified "Open Letter to WHO" by a scientist named Geert Vanden Bossche, claiming mass vaccination would result in severe side effects on the human brain, such as causing Alzheimer's disease.
- *Irrational Behaviors*. Posts on social media about use of garlic to kill the virus triggered irrational garlic consumption by residents in Beijing, Singapore, and Taipei. During the 2020 Chinese New Year, rumors that *shuanghuanglian*, a Chinese herb, could cure COVID-19 led to a buying frenzy (Zhang et al., 2020). In another instance, supermarkets in Hong Kong ran out of toilet paper amid online rumors of a shortage, resulting in panic buying (Caixin, 2020).

These stories are a just small sample of a rising wave of information known as *infodemic* (Cinelli et al., 2020). The term first appeared in 2002 during SARS and refers to "information epidemics" or "epidemics of rumors"— "the rapid spread of information of all kinds, including rumors, gossip, and unreliable information" spread "instantly and internationally" through communication technologies such as mobile phones, social media, and the Internet (World Health Organization, 2020, p. 26).

Infodemics often appear to be mis-, dis-, and mal-information, ranging from rumors, hoaxes, and conspiracy theories to fake news. The COVID-19 infodemic includes all sorts of misleading and factually inaccurate information or outright falsehoods such as the disease's origin, infection channels, cures, treatments, and side effects of the vaccines. As the disease burgeoned in 2020 and 2021, the infodemic spread like a wildfire on social media platforms and interpersonal social networks (Pertwee et al., 2022; Suarez-Lledo & Alvarez-Galvez, 2021).

Infodemics make it hard for the general public "to find trustworthy sources and reliable guidance when they need it," the World Health Organization (2020) complained. Like a virus itself, infodemics can cause public distrust, panic, and fear. Because misinformation does not carry a label as "fake or unchecked information" with a red flag, it presents and circulates as seemingly true but, mixing some true information with false. When shared via posting, forwarding, and reposting on social media platforms, people might perceive a half-truth as true. Further, misinformation may prevail over accurate and scientific information. For instance, in Singapore and Hong Kong, misinformation about vaccines led to citizens' distrust of the vaccines and threatened the success of the governments' COVID-19 mass vaccination programs (Chen et al., 2022).

Psychologically, misinformation about the COVID-19 pandemic is considered harmful because it epidemically prevents people from accessing and processing timely, accurate, and scientific information (Flew, 2021; Ridder, 2021). As stories in China, Hong Kong, Singapore, and Taiwan attest, misinformation about COVID-19 proved more than a nuisance or a harmless hoax; it seems to have exacerbated the public health crisis, hampered the effectiveness of public vaccine campaigns, and eroded public trust in the government and public health authorities.

COVID-19 misinformation can negatively impact individuals (in terms of misbeliefs, emotions, attitudes, knowledge, and protective behaviors) and society (in terms of public compliance; vaccination rates). Research shows the detrimental effects of misinformation on individuals' cognition, emotions, and behaviors, including fear and confusion (Daly & Robinson, 2021; Liu & Huang, 2020), misbeliefs and incorrect knowledge about the pandemic (Kim & Tandoc, 2022; Wei et al., 2022), reluctance in adopting preventive measures (Lee et al., 2020), noncompliance with public health guidelines (Hoffman, 2019), and increased vaccine distrust and vaccine hesitancy (Dror et al., 2020; Pertwee et al., 2022; Zhang et al., 2020). Accordingly, we have focused on misinformation about the COVID-19 pandemic as our study's primary research concern.

Study Objectives

In responding to the urgent need to combat the infodemic by reducing its spread and mitigating the negative impacts, we have conceptualized and executed this interdisciplinary and collaborative project to explore, clarify, and theorize the dynamics of the emergence, diffusion, and consequences of the infodemic during the COVID-19 pandemic. To be specific, we have sought to examine what kinds of debunked misinformation people encountered on social media, and how exposure to the misinformation affected sharing behavior as well as cognitive outcomes (e.g., misinformation beliefs, knowledge of COVID-19) and attitudinal (e.g., anti-vaccine attitudes) and behavioral responses (e.g., countering misinformation).

Furthermore, we have contextualized the study in four Asian societies: Mainland China, Hong Kong, Singapore, and Taiwan. In this way, we have linked the diffusion of infomedic messages on social media and the impacts to the different socio-political systems of these societies. Specifically, we have aimed to achieve these objectives:

- To uncover the emergence and identify the contents and message attributes of misinformation about COVID-19, to delineate the spatiotemporal patterns of the appearance and disappearance of such information online (see details in Chapters 2 and 3).
- To explore the role of access to digital information in society as structural factor in conditioning the exposure and sharing of COVID-19

misinformation on social media, which triggers cognitive, social, and affective processes.

- To theorize the links between exposure to and sharing of COVID-19 misinformation and mechanisms by which people engage in processing the misinformation following exposure, including risk perception during a public health crisis (see Chapters 4–6).
- To examine the real-world consequences of exposure to disinformation in Mainland China (Beijing), Hong Kong, Taiwan (Taipei), and Singapore: How do different digital media environments (access to web-based sources in particular) condition the access, consumption, and impacts of the COVID-19 infodemic? (Chapters 7–11 report key findings).
- To develop perspectives for a key set of Asian societies by employing multiple contexts of cross-societal analyses of how they respond to and cope with COVID-19 misinformation.

Studying COVID Misinformation in Context

To achieve these objectives in examining how the four societies in Asia have dealt with the infodemic in their long-haul fight against the pandemic, we based our decision on the following considerations:

First, these four cities were among the first to be affected by COVID-19 because of their geographical proximity to Wuhan, the origin of the outbreaks in late 2019, and their close economic and social ties with China. The people in those cities also have shared collective memories about experiencing the SARS outbreaks in 2003. Thus, they provide the contexts to examine the complexity of exposure to misinformation about COVID-19 and a variety of cognitive, emotional, and behavioral responses.

Second, although the COVID-19 situation differed substantially in the four cities in 2021 and 2022, the period of this study, Beijing had 1,095 reported cases, with the lowest infection rate (0.05%) and the highest vaccination rate (90%). Singapore reported the highest infection rate (11.44%) with 65,102 confirmed cases, while Taiwan had the lowest vaccination rate of 1.6%. Hong Kong fell in the middle with a 0.16% infection rate and 32.8% full vaccination rate. Nevertheless, people in these cities have endured the world's longest pandemic and strictest control, including shutdowns, mass PCR testing, the most restrictive measures in quarantine rules, and cross-board control (e.g., the zero COVID policy in China). Thus, residents in those cities have a greater dependency on information, online and offline, to stay informed about the updates on pandemic outbreaks and the government's compliance policies in fighting the pandemic.

Third, misinformation about COVID-19 has become a critical issue in these leading cities largely because of their advanced IT developments and saturated smartphone rates, which make it easier for users to distribute and share information, potentially accelerating the spread of falsehoods about COVID-19 on social media. For example, a claim that "5G can transmit the

COVID-19 virus" untruthfully associated China's deployment of 5G mobile networks with the emergence of COVID-19 in Wuhan. Another example, "Asians are more prone to be infected with the COVID-19 virus and die from it than other races." Therefore, a wealth of misinformation surrounding the COVID-19 pandemic invited systematic examination of the patterns of misinformation exposure and dissemination across the four cities, a topic that has been under-researched compared to Western countries (Buchanan & Benson, 2019; Chadwick & Vaccari, 2019; Gerosa et al., 2021; Loomba et al., 2021; Pennycook et al., 2018) and Africa (Madrid-Morales et al., 2021; Wasserman & Madrid-Morales, 2022).

From a research design perspective, the four cities enabled us to pursue cross-societal analyses because they share a common cultural heritage, Confucian values, and a comparable level of development in IT (e.g., high rate of mobile Internet adoption). On the other hand, the four tech-savvy cities differ markedly in terms of socio-political systems and digital information environments. Taipei, Taiwan's capital city of 2.6 million residents, has a fully democratic government; the city-state of Singapore with a population of 5.6 million represents a limited democracy. With 7.5 million residents living in a special administrative region of China, Hong Kong has thrived under a non-democratic but free system. With 21.5 million people residing in China's capital city, Beijing lies under authoritarian rule.

These different political-socio systems produced critical differences in access to digital information, flow of information, and press freedom across the four cities. To us, access matters a great deal because it affects the exposure, perception, and sharing of COVID-19 misinformation on social media. Moreover, as Iyengar et al. (2010) argued, widely accessible information resources help the public acquire fresh information, understand major news topics, and gain knowledge. Thus, when considering each society/city as our unit of analysis, we believe that the significantly varied level of access to digital information in the four cities would shape the process and effects of widely circulated misinformation about COVID-19 and that the variability in exposure to misinformation would lead us to a better understanding of the emergence, diffusion, and impacts of misinformation in multiple social contexts.

A society's information environment for digital communications includes several integral components: hardware (e.g., infrastructure) and software (e.g., apps), and users (Grant & Meadows, 2018). Johnson and Puplampu (2008) called it an "ecological techno-subsystem" that influences users' cognitive growth and social interactions online. As Wei et al. (2022) explained, although the Internet knows no boundary, access to all sorts of information circulated online is subject to the political, cultural, social, and religious conditions of a country. Government censorship—Internet shutdowns, blockages, firewalls—impose significant barriers to the flow of digital information, hindering access to the information.

According to Wei et al. (2022), information accessibility of a society refers to the extent to which citizens can freely seek and acquire a wide range of digital information from web-based resources (e.g., social media platforms, mobile apps) supported by an advanced IT infrastructure and Internet-friendly policies (e.g., free from censorship). This definition entails both hardware (e.g., infrastructure and networks) and software (e.g., civil liberties and diversity), which are essential to make digital information accessible to the public.

Based on the above definition, the four societies differ markedly in access to digital information. Hong Kong and Singapore are the most technologically advanced, where digital information and content in bilingual or multiple languages circulate freely (in terms of linguistic diversity, Singapore has four official languages and Hong Kong is bilingual, while Taipei and Beijing have one official language). Taipei leads the rest of Taiwan in broad-band connectivity through fiber optic, satellite, and 5G networks; press freedom has been rated as the highest among the four cities. In comparison, despite China's growing Internet penetration rate thanks to the diffusion of the smartphone, a great firewall restricts the Chinese people from using global social media platforms such as Google, Facebook, Twitter, and YouTube, as well as international media outlets. Under these circumstances, Beijing showcases what Wei (2009) called a "media-rich" but "information-poor" system due to restrictions on free flow of information online and offline, which results in limited content diversity.

As summarized in Table 1.1, when compared along six factors (e.g., the state of development in information and communications technologies (ICTs), Internet connectivity, Internet censorship, global competitiveness, press freedom, and range of options in official language), digital information and web-based sources are most accessible to Singaporeans and Hongkongers thanks to high global competitiveness, promising ICT developments, multi-lingual media, and high levels of press freedom. Citizens of Taipei can also freely obtain a wide range of web-based information. Digital information online is much less accessible to residents in Beijing because of the great firewall, censorship, and dominance of official media offline and online.

Table 1.1 Components of information accessibility and operationalization in the four cities

	Beijing	Hong Kong	Taipei	Singapore
Ranking in development in ICTs[a]	59 (China)	12	19	1
Internet connectivity[b]	70% (China)	92%	90%	92%
Internet censorship score[c]	2.2	9.7	9.4	7.5
Press freedom ranking[d]	177	80	43	160
Global cities competitiveness ranking[e]	6	7	49	9
# of official languages	1	2	1	4
Overall Ranking	Low	High	Medium	High

Sources: [a](World Economic Forum, 2016), [b](The World Bank, 2020), [c](Vásquez et al., 2021), [d](Reporters Without Borders, 2021), [e](Kearney, 2021).

An Integrative Framework for Studying Diffusion and Impact of Misinformation in Asia

Our past research (Li et al., 2020; Lo et al., 2022; Wei & Lo, 2021; Wei et al., 2022) indicates that digital information accessibility as a macro factor conditions the exposure to COVID-19 misinformation and subsequent impacts. In other words, access to digital information plays the role of a system-level antecedent in affecting the exposure and subsequent processing of the misinformation. We have presented evidence (see Li et al., 2020; Lo et al., 2022) that societal influences tend to prevail over individual differences in affecting citizens' consumption and engagement with digital information because they provide the necessary social conditions in which individuals' information-seeking and processing take place.

In the context of COVID-19, free access to information from web-based sources helps citizens to learn factual and accurate information in a timely manner for subsequent processing and learning. However, citizens must expend greater cognitive efforts to stay informed about the pandemic if needed information is restricted or otherwise unavailable to them. As Trilling and Schoenbach (2013) suggested, under such a circumstance, only people with enthusiasm for fact-checking, ability to reflect, and access to multiple information sources can keep up with updated and accurate information and acquire sufficient knowledge.

Moreover, from the perspective of the classic marketplace of ideas theory (Ingber, 1984), truth will emerge from the competition of ideas in free exchanges of public discourses. Inferior information circulated in the marketplace, such as misinformation or fake news, will lose out to superior information (e.g., truth). In the context of COVID-19, as Wei et al. (2022) have argued, citizens can stay in the know if they have free access to accurate, objective, and fact-checked information to counterbalance misinformation on social media. In such a circumstance, they are less likely to consume misinformation. Empirically, Shirish et al. (2021)'s comparative analyses of data from 72 countries found that media freedom restrained the spread of COVID-related fake news by tolerating pluralism in information diffusion and assuring people's access to fair, factual, and impartial information. They concluded that when people have free access to impartial and factual information, they are less motivated to seek and disseminate unverified non-factual information. As a result, circulation of misinformation decreases, lowering the frequency of people's exposure to misinformation.

On the other hand, in circumstances of limited information accessibility, the fundamental assumption of the marketplace of ideas as a mechanism to weed out falsehood for the benefit of an informed citizenry may not hold (Hofstetter et al., 1999). What is more, restricted access to digital information may be counter-productive, motivating people to seek and consume more content online no matter whether it's true or not, resulting in a greater likelihood of exposure to misinformation from user-generated content on social media (Lo et al., 2022). In sum, the scarcity of pandemic information due to limited access will likely result in consuming more misinformation.

Drawing on the above, our book conceptualizes access to digital information during the COVID-19 pandemic as a societal-level structural factor that shapes the spread of misinformation and leads to broad social impacts (e.g., beliefs, vaccine attitudes, and knowledge). That is, accessibility as a social context holds the key to understanding the reception and viewing of such information, actions that stimulate cognitive reasoning, emotional and behavioral responses. Additionally, in examining the individual-level variables that predict the diffusion process and consequences of COVID-19 misinformation, we pay particular attention to "S" (misinformation about COVID-19 as stimulus), "R" (reasoning, attention to, and elaboration of the misinformation), "O" (orientation, e.g., risk perception) and "R" (cognitive, emotional, and behavioral responses to the misinformation) out of the "the O-R-S-O-R (Orientation-Stimulus-Reasoning-Orientation-Response) framework" (Shah et al., 2007). We believe that these elements capture the critical cognitive, affective, and social processes that underlie people's attitudinal and behavioral responses to the misinformation.

Figure 1.1 shows our proposed model to examine the emergence and diffusion process of misinformation about COVID-19, as well as impacts of exposure to the misinformation. The model integrates digital information accessibility of the four societies (with their different political systems—a societal factor), with individual-level factors that include exposure to and sharing of misinformation, elaboration, perceived influence of misinformation, negative emotions elicited by such information (e.g., fear and anxiety), and behavioral responses to counter the misinformation. We believe that findings of this cross-societal study will deepen the understanding of a key societal factor—access to digital information—that accounts for the level of exposure to and spread of COVID-19 misinformation and differential impacts of the misinformation on citizens' risk perceptions, beliefs, attitudes, and knowledge in the four Asian societies.

Significance of Study

The ongoing COVID-19 pandemic is a global crisis; how to contain the infodemic is an urgent task for policymakers, health authorities, and social media platform operators around the world. Scholarly research on infodemic has increased remarkably over the past three years. However, most research entailed single-country studies, while cross-societal analyses are limited and large-scale multi-level studies are even fewer. In particular, studies exploring societal-level factors that may accelerate or mitigate the spread of the COVID-19 misinformation that amplifies or lowers the adverse effects of exposure to the misinformation are scarce.

By investigating the role of information accessibility in shaping exposure to and sharing of popular COVID-19 misinformation on social media

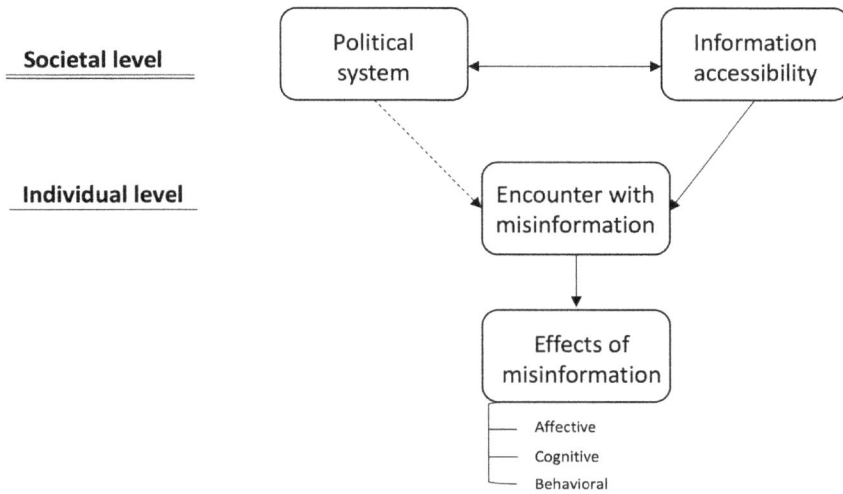

Figure 1.1 An integrated analytic framework of miscommunicating COVID-19

Note: Links in solid lines are relationships examined in this study. Links in dotted lines are theorized relationships but not examined in the study.

platforms that lead to harmful effects on cognitive and attitudinal outcomes (i.e., misinformation beliefs, anti-vaccine attitudes, knowledge of COVID-19), our study of four of Asia's leading cities fills the gap. Findings will lead to insights and generalizations that may be applicable to a wider context beyond the four studied societies. Practically, the findings will provide valuable insights for developing strategies and public policies to contain the "infodemic" on social media channels.

Methodology and Data

The time frame for the fieldwork of this multi-level cross-societal study is tied to the outbreaks of COVID-19 and its variants over the two years of the pandemic during 2021 and 2022. Specifically, the web surveys in Beijing, Hong Kong, Singapore, and Taiwan were conducted in mid-August 2021, when the delta variant of COVID-19 raged across Asia and the rest of the world. Approved COVID-19 vaccines were being promoted globally, but uncertainty and fear about their safety led to anti-vaccine attitudes. The four cities issued strict rules (i.e., quarantines, mass PCR testing, and lockdowns) to control the pandemic. As a result, infection cases were low. By the time of the telephone surveys in July–August 2022 and focus groups in October 2022, the omicron variant hit the four cities, causing the most serious situation with infections numbering in the millions (i.e., Hong Kong, Singapore, and Taipei).

Our cross-societal analysis design goes with a multi-method approach, combining computational big data analytics (i.e., data mining and mathematical modeling) with qualitative and quantitatively social scientific methods (i.e., focus groups and four large-scale surveys). We believe the combined methods will generate different kinds of evidence. The mixture of quantitative and qualitative methods will enable us to triangulate in validating key findings across different methods and across the four societies to draw generalizable conclusions. For instance, focus group discussions will enable us to explore and understand different forms of communication in people's everyday interactions, such as anecdotes, debates, arguments, or even jokes (Green & Thorogood, 2018).

Methodologically, to explore, clarify, and examine the different aspects concerning the emergence, diffusion, and consequences of infodemic messages during the COVID-19 pandemic across the four societies, we adopt a staged design that starts with big data analytics followed by surveys and big data modeling, and ends with focus groups. In this way, each method builds on the proceeding evidence and informs the next. For example, misinformation messages identified in big data analytics are used to construct the survey questionnaire. Findings from parallel surveys are incorporated into mathematical modeling of the diffusion process of such messages. The overview of the design is presented in Table 1.2.

Table 1.2 Research methodology of COVID-19 misinformation

Overview	Emergence ⟶	Diffusion ⟶	Impacts
Big data analytics ⟶	To identify and collect infodemic messages on social media through text mining		
Big data modeling ⟶		To develop a mathematical diffusion model to describe the spreading pattern in online social networks informed by social media data, preliminary surveys.	
Survey ⟶		To measure and analyze variables concerning Exposure-Processing-Consequences (Stimulus-Response-Consequences)	
Focus Group ⟶		To understand why and how people are exposed to, engaged with infomedic messages and counter-measures taken	

Research Methods

Big Data Analytics

To collect popular yet debunked misinformation on social media, we rely on text mining, a big data analytic method, to select the messages concerning the COVID-19 pandemic in two steps. We first aim to collect popular and debunked misinformation from fact-checking websites in the four cities; using keywords search, we search leading social media platforms (i.e., Facebook, Twitter, and Weibo) in each city to confirm that the messages were circulating at the time of study. A list of popular yet debunked misinformation messages is to be generated accordingly (for details, see Chapter 4). Those messages are the centerpiece of our cross-societal analyses as well as the stimuli in designing follow-up surveys and focus group protocols in the four cities.

To further analyze the dynamics of infodemic diffusion on social media during the pandemic, we also use computational methods by virtue of proposing and testing mathematical models to investigate the relationship between social media user characteristics such as location, verification status, the number of followers, and their vulnerability to encountering misinformation. Results will illuminate the pressing questions of who are the most vulnerable and who are the super-spreaders.

Large-Scale Parallel Surveys

In the next step, we develop two types of surveys, web, and telephone, in the four societies to collect data systematically about exposure and attention to debunked disinformation about COVID-19, cognitive reasoning about the infodemic message, perceptions of infodemic messages as a risk as predictors of support for government measures to restrict infodemics, and action to counter disinformation. The survey data also enables us to examine the similarities and differences of respondents in their information processing strategies, perceived risks, and behavioral responses under different conditions of accessibility to digital information.

Modeling the Dynamic Diffusion Process

We use survey results and social media data to build a mathematical diffusion model to describe, clarify, and predict how infodemic messages spread on Weibo in China. The vulnerability of the respondents is assessed in relation to their source characteristics.

Focus Groups

Following the surveys, we conduct focus groups in each city to help better understand why certain groups of people are more prone to encounter or avoid infodemic messages on social media platforms, how their everyday life, including daily routines and coping strategies in dealing with the pandemic, is influenced by infodemics, and what types of counter-measures they have taken to fight the tide of harmful infodemics. Thus, the focus groups provide qualitative in-depth insights and details that complement the quantitative findings.

Data for Analyses

Big Data and COVID-19 Misinformation

Debunked misinformation was collected from fact-checking websites in the four cities, including Tencent Fact (vp.fact.qq.com) based in Beijing, *FactCheck Center* of Taiwan (public@tfc-taiwan.org.tw) and Taiwan-based *MyGo-Pen (mygopen.com)*, Hong Kong-based *Kauyim* (kauyimmedia), the Hong Kong Government News Site (news.gov.hk), Singapore-located *Black Dot Research* (blackdotresearch.sg), and the website of Singapore's Ministry of Health. Debunked messages had to appear in at least two of the cities to be included. These selected messages are then searched by keywords on leading social media platforms such as Weibo, Facebook, and Twitter to check whether they were circulating. A list of popular yet debunked misinformation messages is made using these procedures. The list of COVID-19 misinformation messages text mined for the study is available in Appendix 1.A.

Survey Data

Online parallel surveys were conducted to collect data in Beijing, Hong Kong, Taipei, and Singapore from August 4 to 18, 2021. The fieldwork protocol was approved by the Institutional Review Board. To randomly select respondents, a national panel was used with an email invitation to complete a web-based survey. We used standardized measures and scales for key constructs of the study. Details of the operationalization of the independent and dependent variables are provided in each chapter. The questionnaire was administered in traditional Chinese in Hong Kong and Taipei, in English in Singapore, and in simplified Chinese in Beijing. A total of 4,094 respondents successfully completed the surveys.

Among the 4,094 respondents, the average age was 40.36 (SD = 13.14, ranging from 18 to 84). Of the sample, gender was evenly distributed, consisting of 48.30% males and 51.70% females. The distribution of gender and age basically matched the general population of each city. In terms of educational background, 18.10% respondents received high-school level education or lower, 19.20% held a diploma in vocational education, 52.70% obtained a bachelor's degree, and 10% had a master's degree or higher. Considering that Singapore is a multi-ethnic society, ethnicity in the Singapore sample was measured. The sample included 74% Chinese, 13.70% Malay, 7.60% Indian, and 4.70% other. Appendix 1.B presents the sample profile by site of study.

In addition, four similar parallel telephone surveys were conducted from July 20 to August 30, 2022, a period in which outbreaks of omicron, a variant of COVID-19, were the main concern. The targeted sample size was 1,000 for each city, with 95% confidence interval and ±3.01% sampling error. Data collection in each city was outsourced to professional research institutions or survey companies. RDD was used in generating samples by contracted survey companies in each city. In each city, a database of phone numbers was generated by the combination of area codes and random numbers programmed by a computer. The dialed numbers were chosen randomly from the database. The questionnaire was administered in traditional Chinese in Hong Kong and Taipei, in English in Singapore, and in simplified Chinese in Beijing. A total of 4,114 persons were successfully interviewed. Response rates vary across the four cities but they are consistent with the prevailing rate in each city. Using AAPOR's standard in calculating response rate (Formula 3), the response rates are respectively: 43.0% in Singapore, 55.9% in Taipei, 38.6% in Hong Kong, and 2.2% in Beijing.

Among the 4,114 respondents, the average age was 47.03 (SD = 15.96, ranging from 18 to 94). Of the sample, gender was evenly distributed, consisting of 48.90% males and 51.10% females, matching the distribution of the general populations of each city. In terms of the educational background, 32.80% respondents received high-school level education or lower, 20.20% held a diploma in vocational education, 36.0% obtained a bachelor's degree, and 11.0% had a master's degree or higher. Appendix 1.C presents the sample profile.

The majority of the chapters in our book (i.e., Chapters 4–9 and 11) rely on the web survey data for analyses; while the data from telephone surveys was used for Chapter 10 on information fatigue during the pandemic.

Focus Groups

Data collection was outsourced to an international data company, Ipsos. In total, we recruited 80 participants. They were selected by age (20ish–40ish as younger vs. 40ish–60ish as older) and level of encounters with misinformation related to COVID-19 (avoiding COVID-19 information vs. encountering COVID-19 information). Accordingly, there are four mixed groups in each city with each group of five participants. The respondents ranged in age from 21 to 58. Forty-one were male and thirty-nine were female. Their most frequently used social media platforms included Facebook, Instagram, Line, WeChat, Telegram, and WhatsApp.

A framework of structured discussion guide was developed based on the key findings from the large-scale surveys; it focused on the encounter and engagement with the same false or fact-checked inaccurate or unscientific messages used in the web surveys. Appendix 1.D has the framework for developing fieldwork protocols. The 16 online sessions of the focus groups were convened in October 2022, with each session lasting for 1.5 hours.

Discussions were moderated by a professional moderator. See the detailed protocol in Appendix 1.E. The data and insights from focus groups are used in the book to complement the quantitative findings.

Outline of the Book

What to expect next? This team-authored book consists of three sections: (1) introduction and foundations, (2) the process and impacts of misinformation COVID-19, and (3) conclusions and insights.

Chapters 2 and 3 identify and trace the emergence and diffusion of misinformation on social media surrounding COVID-19 in the four studied societies. The spatial patterns and attributes of such messages are presented. What kinds of COVID-19 misinformation do people encounter on popular social media platforms? How do these messages spread online? When and how? Who is the source and who is the most vulnerable? Chapters 4 and 5 analyze exposure to and sharing of popular yet debunked COVID-19 misinformation messages identified in the previous two chapters.

The next four chapters (Chapters 6–8) examine the predictors and mechanisms that lead to adverse effects of exposure to COVID-19 misinformation (e.g., misbeliefs, attitudes, trust, knowledge, and counteractions). Chapter 9 concerns the public's information overload and avoidance during the long-haul pandemic as a result of exposure to misinformation about COVID-19. The next chapter, Chapter 10, explores the public's actions to fight back misinformation, including demographic characteristics of those who take various types of actions against falsehood and predictors of those actions. Chapter 11 presents the results of moderation and mediation analyses of the role of moderators and mediators in affecting the processes and adverse effects of pandemic misinformation through theorized pathways. Our conceptual models are validated with evidence. Finally, Chapter 12 draws conclusions and insights that lead to an Asian perspective in combating COVID-19 misinformation.

References

Buchanan, T., & Benson, V. (2019). Spreading disinformation on Facebook: Do trust in message source, risk propensity, or personality affect the organic reach of "fake news"? *Social Media + Society, 5*(4), 1–9. https://doi.org/10.1177/2056305119888654

Caixin. (2020, February 17). *Public panic buying in Hong Kong.* https://china.caixin.com/2020-02-17/101516388.html

Chadwick, A., & Vaccari, C. (2019). *News sharing on UK social media: Misinformation, disinformation, and correction.* Online Civic Culture Centre, Loughborough University. https://repository.lboro.ac.uk/articles/report/News_sharing_on_UK_social_media_misinformation_disinformation_and_correction/9471269

Chen, K., Chen, A., Zhang, J., Meng, J., & Shen, C. (2020). Conspiracy and debunking narratives about COVID-19 origins on Chinese social media: How it started and who is to blame. *Harvard Kennedy School (HKS) Misinformation Review, 1*(8), 1–30. https://doi.org/10.37016/mr-2020-50

Chen, X., Lee, W., & Lin, F. (2022). Infodemic, institutional trust, and COVID-19 vaccine hesitancy: A cross-national survey. *International Journal of Environmental Research and Public Health, 19*(13), 8033. https://doi.org/10.3390/ijerph19138033

Cinelli, M., Quattrociocchi, W., Galeazzi, A., Valensise, C., Brugnoli, E., Schmidt, A., Zola, P., Zollo, F., & Scala, A. (2020). The COVID-19 social media infodemic. *Scientific Reports, 10*, 16598. https://doi.org/10.1038/s41598-020-73510-5

Daly, M., & Robinson, E. (2021). Willingness to vaccinate against COVID-19 in the US: Representative longitudinal evidence from April to October 2020. *American Journal of Preventive Medicine, 60*(6), 766–773. https://doi.org/10.1016/j.amepre.2021.01.008

Dror, A. A., Eisenbach, N., Taiber, S., et al. (2020). Vaccine hesitancy: The next challenge in the fight against COVID-19. *European Journal of Epidemiology, 35*, 775–779. https://doi.org/10.1007/s10654-020-00671-y

Flew, T. (2021). The global trust deficit disorder: A communications perspective on trust in the time of global pandemics. *Journal of Communication, 71*(2), 163–186. https://doi.org/10.1093/joc/jqab006

Gerosa, T., Gui, M., Hargittai, E., & Nguyen, M. H. (2021). (Mis) informed during COVID-19: How education level and information sources contribute to knowledge gaps. *International Journal of Communication, 15*, 2196–2217. https://ijoc.org/index.php/ijoc/article/view/16438

Grant, A., & Meadows, J. (2018). *Communication technology update and fundamentals* (14th edition). NY: Focal Press.

Green, J., & Thorogood, N. (2018). *Qualitative methods for health research*. sage.

Hamilton, I. A. (2020, May 6). 77 cell phone towers have been set on fire so far due to a weird coronavirus 5G conspiracy theory. *Business Insider*. https://www.businessinsider.in/ tech/news/77-cell-phone-towers-have-been-set-on-fire-so-far-due-to-a-weird-coronavirus-5g-conspiracy-theory/articleshow/75580457.cms

Hoffman, J. (2019, September 23). How anti-vaccine sentiment took hold in the United States. *The New York Times*. https://www.nytimes.com/2019/09/23/health/anti-vacci- nation-movement-us.html

Hofstetter, C. R., Barker, D., Smith, J. T., Zari, G. M., & Ingrassia, T. A. (1999). Information, misinformation, and political talk radio. *Political Research Quarterly, 52*(2), 353–369. https://doi.org/10.2307/449222

Ingber, S. (1984). The marketplace of ideas: A legitimizing myth. *Duke Law Journal, 1*(3), 1–91.

Iyengar, S., Curran, J., Lund, A. B., Salovaara-Moring, I., Hahn, K. S., & Coen, S. (2010). Cross-national versus individual-level differences in political information: A media systems perspective. *Journal of Elections, Public Opinion and Parties, 20*(3), 291–309. https://doi.org/10.1080/17457289.2010.490707

Johnson, G. M., & Puplampu, K. P. (2008). Internet use during childhood and the ecological techno-subsystem. *Canadian Journal of Learning and Technology, 34*(1), n1. https://doi.org/10.21432/T2CP4T

Kearney. (2021). *2021 Global Cities Report*. https://www.kearney.com/global-cities/2021

Kim, H., & Tandoc, Jr., E. (2022). Consequences of online misinformation on COVID-19: Two potential pathways and disparity by eHealth literacy. *Frontiers in Psychology, 13*, 1–10. https://doi.org/10.3389/fpsyg.2022.783909

Lee, J. J., Kang, K.-A., Wang, M. P., Zhao, S. Z., Wong, J. Y. H., O'Connor, S., Yang, S. C., & Shin, S. (2020, 2020/11/13). Associations between COVID-19 misinformation exposure and belief with COVID-19 knowledge and preventive behaviors: Cross-sectional online study. *Journal Medical Internet Research*, 22(11), e22205. https://doi.org/10.2196/22205

Li, Z., Lo, V., Wei, R., Zhang, G., & Chen, Y. (2020). The impact of mobile news use, need for orientation and information environment on political knowledge. *Journalism Research, 7*, 105–120.

Liu, P. L., & Huang, L. V. (2020). Digital disinformation about COVID-19 and the third-person effect: Examining the channel differences and negative emotional outcomes. *Cyberpsychology, Behavior, and Social Networking, 23*(11), 789–793. https://doi.org/10.1089/cyber.2020.0363

Lo, V., Wei, R., Lu, M., Zhang, X., & Qiu, J. L. (2022, May 20–26). *A comparative study of the impact of digital media environments, information processing and presumed influence on behavioral responses to COVID-19 misinformation in four Asian cities* [Paper presentation]. 2022 International Communication Association Annual Conference, Paris, France.

Loomba, S., de Figueiredo, A., Piatek, S. J., de Graaf, K., & Larson, H. J. (2021). Measuring the impact of COVID-19 vaccine misinformation on vaccination intent in the UK and USA. *Nature Human Behaviour, 5*(3), 337–348. https://doi.org/10.1038/s41562-021-01056-1

Madrid-Morales, D., Wasserman, H., Gondwe, G., Ndlovu, K., Sikanku, E., Tully, M., ... Uzuegbunam, C. (2021). Motivations for sharing misinformation: A comparative study in six Sub- Saharan African countries. *International Journal of Communication, 15*, 20. https://ijoc.org/index.php/ijoc/article/view/14801

Pennycook, G., Cannon, T. D., & Rand, D. G. (2018). Prior exposure increases perceived accuracy of fake news. *Journal of Experimental Psychology: General, 147*(12), 1865–1880. https://doi.org/10.1037/xge0000465

Pertwee, E., Simas, C., & Larson, H. J. (2022). An epidemic of uncertainty: Rumors, conspiracy theories and vaccine hesitancy. *Nature Medicine, 28*, 456–459. https://doi.org/10.1038/s41591-022-01728-z

Reporters Without Borders. (2021). *World Press Freedom Index 2021*. https://rsf.org/en/index?year=2021

Ridder, J. (2021). What's so bad about misinformation? *Inquiry*, 1–23. https://doi.org/10.1080/0020174X.2021.2002187

Shah, D., Cho, J., Nah, S., Gotlieb, M., Hwang, H., Lee, N., ... McLeod, D. (2007). Campaign ads, online messaging, and participation: Extending the communication mediation model. *Journal of Communication, 57*(4), 676–703. https://doi.org/10.1111/j.1460-2466.2007.00363.x

Shirish, A., Srivastava, S. C., & Chandra, S. (2021). Impact of mobile connectivity and freedom on fake news propensity during the COVID-19 pandemic: A cross-country empirical examination. *European Journal of Information Systems, 30*(3), 322–341. https://doi.org/10.1080/0960085X.2021.1886614

Suarez-Lledo, V., & Alvarez-Galvez, J. (2021). Prevalence of health misinformation on social media: Systematic review. *Journal of Medical Internet Research, 23*, e17187. https://doi.org/10.2196/17187. https://www.jmir.org/2021/1/e17187

The World Bank. (2020). *Individuals using the Internet (% of the population)*. https://data.worldbank.org/indicator/IT.NET.USER.ZS

Trilling, D., & Schoenbach, K. (2013). Skipping current affairs: The non-users of online and offline news. *European Journal of Communication, 28*(1), 35–51. https://doi.org/10.1177/0267323112453671

Vásquez, I., McMahon, F., Murphy, R., & Sutter Schneider, G. (2021). *Human Freedom Index 2021*. Cato Institute and Fraser Institute. https://www.cato.org/human-freedom-index/2021

Wasserman, H., & Madrid-Morales, D. (2022). *Disinformation in the Global South*. Hoboken, NJ: John Wiley & Sons, Inc. https://doi.org/10.1002/9781119714491

Wei, R. (2009). The state of new media technology research in China: A review and critique. *Asian Journal of Communication, 19*(1), 115–126. https://doi.org/10.1080/01292980802603991

Wei, R., & Lo, V.-H. (2021). *News in their pockets*. Oxford University Press.

Wei, R., Guo, J., Wang, S., & Huang, Y. (2022). The role of digital information accessibility in shaping the relationships of exposure to COVID-19 misinformation and cognitive and attitudinal effects in Asia. *Communication & Society, 62*, 127–159. http://www.cschinese.com/issueArticle.asp?P_No=93&CA_ID=708

World Economic Forum. (2016). *The Global Information Technology Report 2016*. https://www.weforum.org/reports/the-global-information-technology-report-2016/

World Health Organization. (2020). *Infodemic*. World Health Organization. https://www.who.int/health-topics/infodemic#tab=tab_1

Zhang, L., Chen, K., Jiang, H., & Zhao, J. (2020). How the health rumor misleads people's perception in a public health emergency: Lessons from a purchase craze during the COVID-19 outbreak in China. *International Journal of Environmental Research and Public Health, 17*(19), 1–15. https://doi.org/10.3390/ijerph17197213

2 The Emergence of COVID-19 Misinformation
Conception and Message Characteristics

Hai Liang, Ran Wei, and Anfan Chen

Misinformation about COVID-19 Defined

A hallmark of the COVID-19 pandemic has been the rising tide of misinformation—information that is false, factually incorrect, or misleading concerning various aspects of the virus. Although the taxonomies of false, inaccurate, or misleading information about COVID-19 have expanded to dis- and mal-information or fake news, to the best of our knowledge, there is no such comprehensive and conclusive definition of misinformation. For example, in computational social science, misinformation refers to incorrect or misleading messages (Lazer et al., 2018). This definition has been criticized as problematic because it leads to inaccurate beliefs and greater disagreement over specific aspects of the information (e.g., truth, reliability, verifiability).

Our study focuses on COVID-19 misinformation, which differs from disinformation and mal-information. According to documents compiled by UNESCO (2018, p. 7), misinformation refers to information that is misleading but created or disseminated "without manipulative or malicious intent." As Southwell et al. (2018, p. 1) suggested, such information can be "deliberately promoted and accidentally shared" online. Disinformation, on the other hand, is orchestrated information that deliberately attempts to cause confusion or manipulate the public for economic or political gains, whereas mal-information refers to information that is true but weaponized to harm a targeted individual or institution.

Misinformation also differs from fake news in terms of the format of presentation and style. Misinformation is commonly presented as posted or blogged claims on social media, while fake news is typically presented in the form of news reports with a headline, lead, text, and accompanying photo or graphics. In the political context, Nyhan and Reifler (2010, p. 305) defined misinformation as "the presence of objectively incorrect or false information, which is not supported by clear evidence and expert opinion." Kim and Tandoc (2022) expanded the term to claims that have been debunked or corrected by expert scientific consensus that is either completely false or misleading.

DOI: 10.4324/9781003355984-2

Based on the above review, we conceptualize COVID-19 misinformation as unverified messages that contain false claims or factually incorrect information about COVID-19 that appear to be scientifically based. We call it "specious information" in Chinese ("似是而非的資訊"). In other words, we view misinformation concerning the COVID-19 pandemic as something like half-truths, a mixture of true, scientific information with false, incorrect claims or assertions without proven evidence. For example, BCG (Bacillus Calmette–Guérin vaccine) protects against the coronavirus; alcohol kills the virus. In other cases, assertions portray some claims as being absolutely correct. Take the misinformation on the origin of the virus as an example.

Operationally, as Kim and Tandoc (2022) argued, deciding what is scientifically true or false in a claim is complicated due to the inherent uncertainty of science. Likewise, spotting and classifying COVID-19 misinformation is also challenging and beyond the scope of our study. For instance, labeling a message as misinformation may cause concern about threats to civic freedoms, freedom of the press, and outright censorship, among others. In this chapter, instead of attempting to classify information about COVID-19 on social media, we take the combined approach of data mining analytics with manual content analyses: First, we collect a set of infodemic messages that had been identified by professional fact-checking websites or organizations; second, we integrate manual and computer-assisted content analysis to obtain a keyword list, which was frequently used to correct/refute/debunk online falsehood, and proved to be an effective instrumental in identifying infodemic messages in our dataset.

The Emergence and Topical Trends of COVID-19 Misinformation on Weibo

Since January 2020 when the COVID-19 pandemic broke out, popular social media platforms made the presence of COVID-19 misinformation prevalent in China (Chen et al., 2020; Yang et al., 2021). For instance, prominent misinformation narratives circulated widely on social media platforms. These included unsubstantiated claims about the origins of the virus; whether it was intended to be a bioweapon; and whether Bill Gates engineered the virus for profit. Although the government, news media, and social media platform operators have made intensive efforts to dispel and correct falsehoods, a large amount of misinformation still circulating on Chinese social media (Chen, 2022).

In this chapter, for practical considerations about data accessibility in all of the four cities in our study, we use large-scale datasets from Sina Weibo (hereafter as Weibo), China's most popular Twitter-like micro-messaging site, to assess the emergence and prevalence of misinformation and then examine its temporal-spatial patterns, sources, and content features. The Beijing-headquartered Weibo is a commercial site run by Sina Corporation; its micro-blogging service is accessible to the general public worldwide for self-publishers (e.g., blogging or content creators). As China's political center, cultural center, and IT center, Beijing is the world's most populous capital city. More than 21 million residents live in the capital city, where social media users from all walks of life concentrate.

Procedurally, a few misinformation-identification approaches have been developed to examine information authenticity either automatically (i.e., based on computer processing) or manually (i.e., based on human judgment, such as experts or platforms. see Zhou & Zafarani, 2020). At least four types of approaches have been proposed to detect online misinformation (Allen et al., 2021; Grinberg et al., 2019; Zhou & Zafarani, 2020):

1 **knowledge-based approach,** which detects misinformation by judging if the referred knowledge in the message (text) is consistent with facts. For example, comparing the knowledge extracted from to-be-verified news content with known facts, with experts or crowd-sources fact-checking methods;
2 **style-based approach,** showing how the information is formatted and framed. Malicious entities prefer to write "fake" news in a special style to encourage others to read and convince them to trust, such as exaggeration and swearing;
3 **network-based approach,** mapping the misinformation by how it's spread and how actors are connected online, such as investigating and using the information related to the dissemination of false messages;
4 **source-based approach,** evaluating the credibility of information sources or citations.

In this study, we mixed the knowledge-based approach with the expert fact-checking method in detecting the emergence of misinformation about COVID-19 on Weibo.

Findings

The Emergence of Misinformation about COVID-19 on Weibo

To estimate the emergence, prevalence, and temporal-spatial patterns of COVID-19 misinformation, we collect data from Weibo, which has 560 million monthly active users (Sina Weibo, 2021). The advanced search function of Weibo, as well as a list of representative keywords manually summarized from 2,970 COVID-19 misinformation cases from two Chinese fact-checking websites—Tencent Jiaozhen (news.qq.com/Original/jzhjym. htm) and Weibo Piyao (weibo.com/weibopiyao), are implemented in retrieving COVID-19 misinformation-related posts on Weibo published between January 1, 2020 and February 6, 2022. After removing duplicates, we obtain a total of 285,695 original posts published by 81,829 unique users.

All posts are retrieved using misinformation-related keywords, including those that debunked misleading or false posts. To filter out debunking posts, we manually summarize 34 seed keywords that are related to debunking narratives, such as "rumor," "don't believe," "fake," "not true," "conspiracy," and "spread the truth" (for the full list, see Appendix 2.A). Using a method called "word embeddings" (Garg et al., 2018; Kroon et al., 2021) and a pre-trained word embeddings model by Tencent AI Lab (Tencent, 2022), we expand the initial list to 399 keywords that are semantically correlated and similar to the seed words. To validate the performance of the keyword-based classification method, we randomly sample 1,000 posts and manually code if a post is debunking or misinformation. The results show that the keyword-based approach has achieved a satisfactory performance, with an agreement with human annotation of Krippendorff's alpha coefficient at 0.786. Accordingly, our dataset includes 192,542 misinformation posts (posted by 61,700 users) and 93,423 debunking posts (posted by 20,129 users).

Figure 2.1 presents the temporal trends of all misinformation posts between 2020 and 2022, from which several trends emerged. First, most misinformation messages were posted at the early stage of the pandemic in 2020 and the number of posts declined gradually over the following six months. Second, several peaks can be observed, which coincided with different waves of COVID-19 outbreaks: Phase 1 between January 29, 2020 and April 9, 2020 (initial outbreaks of Delta virus, a variant of SARS-CoV-2, in China),

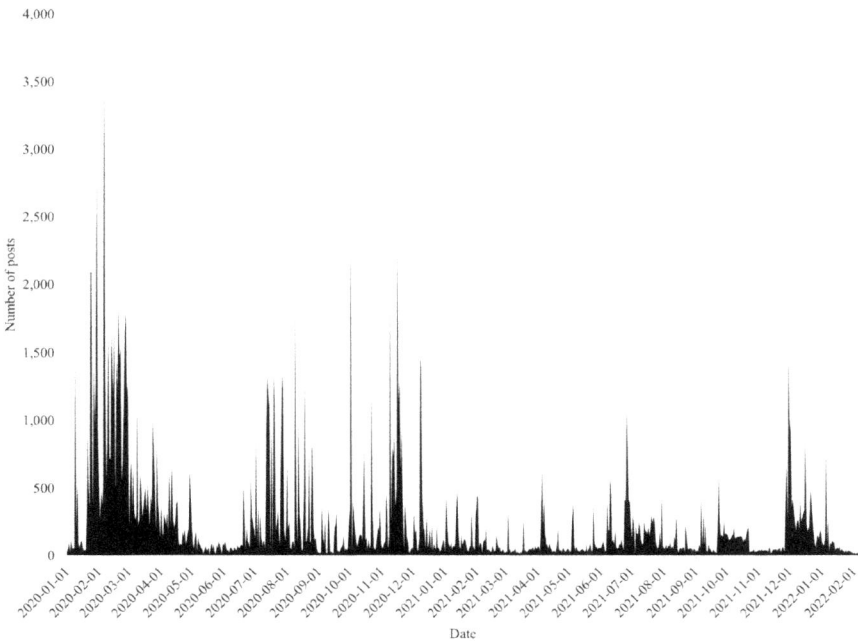

Figure 2.1 Time series of emergence of identified Weibo posts pertaining to COVID-19 misinformation

Phase 2 between June 20, 2020 and September 11, 2020 (the first wave in the United States), Phase 3 between October 2, 2020 and February 1, 2021 (2020 United States presidential election), and Phase 4 between November 28, 2021 and January 5, 2022 (Omicron, another variant of SARS-CoV-2, uprising with a global outbreak).

Topics of COVID-19 Misinformation Posts on Weibo

To categorize the collected posts, we adopt topic modeling to detect the hidden topics that emerge from a large collection of posts. Specifically, we conducted a Latent Dirichlet allocation (i.e., LDA) model (Blei, 2012) on all collected posts. Based on the results of the LDA modeling process, we chose the optimal k value of 30 topics for our model. Then, the automatically generated keywords of the 30 topics were read carefully and labeled by a native Chinese speaker and communication expert. Finally, we manually recoded the 30 extracted topics into 13 topical frames (see Appendix 2.B).

As presented in Figure 2.2, among all original posts related to COVID-19 misinformation, the most prevalent topics are concerned with the origin of COVID-19 (23.63%), publicity such as government announcements or updates on the outbreaks (16.68%), and prevention measures such as compliance (9.15%), followed by vaccination (8.67%), quarantine policies

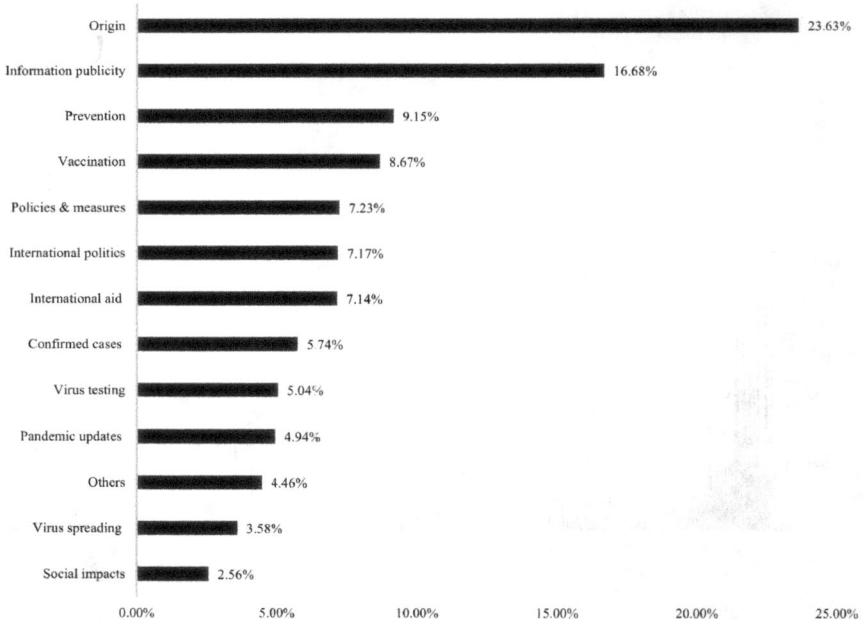

Figure 2.2 Distribution of posts of COVID-19 misinformation message by topical categories (N = 285,695)

and measures (7.23%), international aspects of the pandemic (7.17%), international aid (7.14%), daily confirmed cases (5.74%), virus testing (5.04%), updates on pandemic variants (4.94%), virus spreading (3.58%), and the social impacts of the pandemic (2.56%). The rest, coded as "other," account for 4.46%. The topical features of Weibo seem to be more diverse and wide-ranging compared to other studies (e.g., Zeng & Chan, 2021) which reported that the most prevailing topics in Chinese pieces of misinformation were about travel restrictions and travelers who spread the virus.

The topics of misinformation over the two years are matched with the timeline of the outburst of posts on Weibo. The evolving trends of ups and downs in topics are shown in Figure 2.3. The origin of COVID-19 is a recurring topic and the proportion generally increased over the entire period of two years. Additionally, among the most posted topics, misinformation about preventive measures is more consistent while misinterpretation or faulty posting on official publicity (e.g., updates, daily briefings, and policy announcements) decreases over time.

Sources of Misinformation on Weibo

Because all Weibo posts we collect are original after excluding reposts, we consider the users who posted the misinformation messages (e.g.,

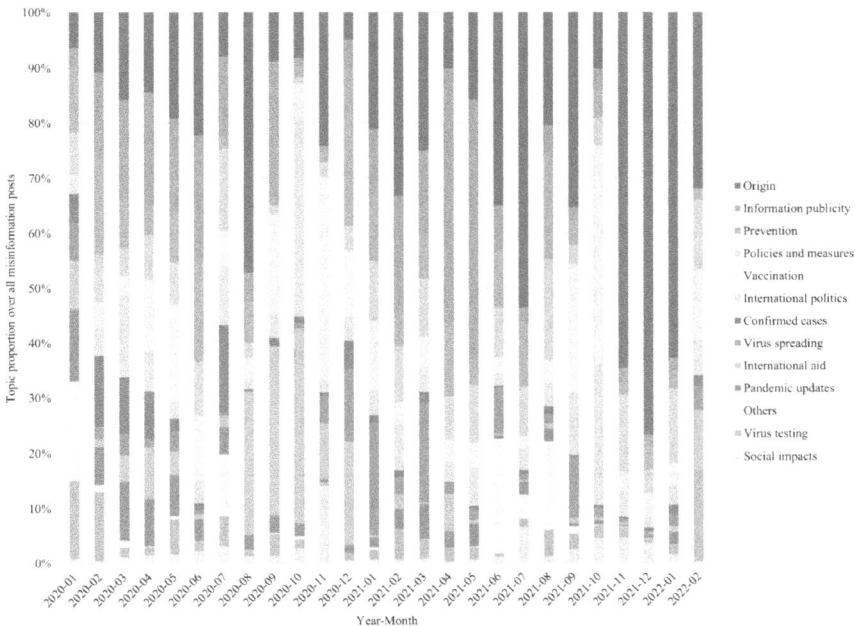

Figure 2.3 Time distribution of posts of COVID-19 misinformation message by categories

bloggers, content creators, or content curators) as a proxy of the source of misinformation according to the categories of account they hold: (1) government accounts, including a variety of departments and branches of the Chinese government at all levels from national to village-level; (2) media accounts, including all sorts of media organizations, professional journalists, editors, and TV hosts/hostess, and web-based freelancers such as bloggers, publishers or self-appointed hosts; (3) verified individual users (aka influential content creators), those who actively create information for others to consume and whose identities have been verified by Weibo; (4) corporation accounts, including accounts affiliated to commercial entities; and (5) unverified individual users (e.g., the rest, which is the majority of Weibo users).

As Table 2.1 shows, most of the misinformation sources are ordinary individual account holders who were either anonymous or whose identities were not verified. They account for nearly two-thirds of the sources of posted COVID-19 misinformation on Weibo (60.58%), followed by verified individual account holders (23.81%). The rest are sourced by holders or creators of government accounts (7.54%), corporation accounts (5.58%), and media accounts (2.49%).

Although the two types of individual account holders proportionally account for 84.39% of all misinformation sources, they only generate 52.92% of misinformation messages. Surprisingly, government and media account holders have posted 40.96% of misinformation messages. In a closer look at these sources, we note that the majority of those government accounts are run by local governments at the grassroots (e.g., township party committee or party secretary of a village). The high percentage of misinformation posted from those accounts suggests that the local government account holders may lack the know-how in filtering pandemic information and sorting out infodemic messages. Similarly, a great number of media accounts are created and operated by so-called free-lance content creators, not the official media. They are sources of misinformation because they may be either misled by falsehoods or motivated by business incentives to unintentionally or intentionally promote misinformation messages.

In addition, self-reported gender can be directly retrieved from Weibo profile, with 1 = male (n = 195,922, 68.58%), and 0 = female (n = 89,773,

Table 2.1 Posted misinformation messages about COVID-19 by types of sources (n = 61,700)

Account types	N (%) of accounts	N (%) of posts
Ordinary individual account	37,376 (60.58%)	60,045 (31.19%)
Verified individual account	14,689 (23.81%)	41,832 (21.73%)
Government account	4,653 (7.54%)	41,230 (21.42%)
Corporation account	3,444 (5.58%)	11,795 (6.13%)
Media account	1,538 (2.49%)	37,607 (19.54%)
Total	61,700 (100%)	192,509 (100%)

31.42%). Based on the profile information, we also obtain the number of followers (M = 10,297, Mdn = 8,966, SD = 2,305), the number of followees (those who are followed by the engaged user) (M = 667, Mdn = 297, SD = 1,382), and the number of historical posts (M = 10,518, Mdn = 2,924, SD = 115,487) for each engaged user in our dataset. The results of these additional analyses suggest that male users were more likely to post misinformation posts than were female users (male = 33.30%, female = 27.50%), while female users were more likely to be associated with debunking posts than were male users (female = 72.50%, male = 66.70%), with a significant difference, χ^2 (1, N = 285,695) = 962.089, p < .001. Verified accounts were less likely to post misinformation than debunking messages (66.90% vs. 78.40%), while unverified accounts were more likely to post misinformation than debunking messages (33.10% vs. 21.60%), with a significant difference, χ^2 (1, N = 285,695) = 3,971.300, p < .001. However, we did not find any significant differences in terms of the number of followers, followees, or historical posts of users.

Characteristics of Misleading COVID-19 Messages

Some textual features are extracted from the Weibo posts and have been examined in previous social media studies. Factors have included the length of the texts and whether the posts include pictures, hashtags, or URLs. We used existing tools to extract other latent features. For example, the emotion score of each post was calculated based on the methods by Zhang et al. (2017) and Liu (2010). To be specific, positive words were assigned the value equal to +1, while negative words with –1. The emotion scores of positive and negative words were adjusted in the case of transition words (e.g., but). The emotion score was also adjusted by weighting for each polarity score according to its adverbs of degree. To complete the calculation, the valence of each polarity word in a post was added to obtain an emotion score for each post.

A larger value indicates more positive emotions. The detection of uncivil posts is based on the word embedding method and a pre-trained word embedding model by Tencent AI Lab (Tencent, 2022). Specifically, we developed a list of 2,643 uncivil words from a list of 40 seed uncivil words obtained from Song et al. (2021).

Since the abovementioned variables were proposed to examine social media texts in general, they might not be specific to misinformation. We also compared the features of misinformation messages with debunking messages to see what features might be related to misinformation messages.

As Table 2.2 shows, in terms of message attributes, 36.60% of the messages included a picture, 64.50% carried hashtags, and only 0.64% included hyperlinks, suggesting most misinformation messages did not have a clear source. Nevertheless, they were the common features of social media posts related to COVID-19, at least on Weibo. Interestingly, one-third (33.05%)

Table 2.2 Content features of misinformation and debunking messages

	Misinformation	Debunking
	N (%)	N (%)
Pictures	70,455 (36.6%)	45,850 (49.1%)
Hashtag	124,196 (64.5%)	64,330 (68.8%)
URL	1,233 (0.64%)	255 (0.27%)
Uncivil words	63,632 (33.05%)	19,327 (20.68%)
	M (Mdn, SD)	M (Mdn, SD)
Emotion intensity	12.38 (7.86, 25.80)	10.35 (6.88, 23.40)
Text length	199.80 (146.0, 295.80)	229.60 (145.00, 360.90)

of the misinformation messages used uncivil words such as vulgarity and swearing. In addition, they were more emotional. Compared to debunking messages, misinformation messages were more likely to include positive emotions (12.38 vs. 10.35, $t = 21.0$, $p < .001$) and uncivil words (33.05% vs. 20.68%, χ^2 (1, N = 285,695) = 1,706.3, $p < .001$), but more likely to be shorter (199.80 vs. 229.60, $t = 21.9$, $p < .001$). These unique features of misinformation indicate that misinformation can be more eye-catching and thus spread more widely than debunking and other messages as indicated in previous studies (e.g., Vosoughi et al., 2018).

Summary of Key Findings

In summary, using big data from Weibo and computational methods and with a focus on temporal and topical distribution, source, and message characteristics, a number of patterns of COVID-19 misinformation were uncovered in the present chapter:

- Most misinformation messages were posted at the early stage of the pandemic in 2020 and the number of posts declined gradually over the following six months.
- Several peaks in posting were observed, which coincided with different waves of COVID-19 outbreaks. That is, whenever there was a new outbreak, posting concerning COVID-19 that was half truths or total falsehood would increase in largest numbers.
- Misinformation concerning the COVID-19 appeared to be shorter, with no URLs, and more attractive in visual appeal crafted for wider reach on social media.
- The origin of COVID-19 was the most prevalent topic, followed by false messages about updates on the pandemic and compliance measures.
- In terms of sources, ordinary individual and male users accounted for most of the posted misinformation, whereas institutional and female users were more likely to post debunking information.

Implications

In this chapter, we have applied computational methods to analyze a set of massive social media corpus collected from Weibo in Beijing for two years to sketch out the emergence of misinformation surrounding COVID-19 and assess its temporal and topical features in terms of trending patterns, prevailing topics, sources, and content features of the misinformation. The following is a summary of our key findings:

First, temporal patterns of misinformation posts on Weibo show that falsehoods about COVID-19 started with a burst and then increased rapidly with several peaks, and that this pattern repeated periodically. Specifically, our data found that 5 out of 13 topics on COVID-19 misinformation resurged multiple times. Temporal recurrence of such misinformation messages and the recurring spread of misinformation may hinder falsehood spreaders from strategically keeping false rumors alive in hopes of influencing followers or followees. This finding lends critical implications for misinformation correction practices by authorities and medical agencies: countering the infodemic could not be accomplished with a single campaign. Persistent efforts are needed to counter or correct misinformation during and ever after a pandemic.

Second, the most posted topics of misinformation messages are about the original COVID-19, information publicity, and compliance. These findings are comparable to the previous study by Chen et al. (2020), indicating that the origination of COVID-19 was the locus of public attention in the infodemic. Although the top three topics were also the most prevalent in debunking messages, we observed significant differences in topics between posting misinformation and debunking messages. Even though 23.63% of misinformation posts were about COVID-19 origin, only 11.94% of debunking messages were related to the topic. On the contrary, 9.36% of debunking messages were about the virus spreading, and only 3.58% were misinformation related to it. This is especially critical in terms of the misinformation countering effectiveness, since this type of divergence and mismatch may temper the efficiency of misinformation correction efforts enacted by multiple users.

Third, individual accounts, no matter verified or not, tend to post more misinformation than debunking messages, whereas government and media accounts were more likely to post debunking than misinformation messages. Nevertheless, government and media accounts also posted more than 40% of misinformation messages in total. As the Chinese public relies heavily on social media channels for updated information and social interactions to cope with the COVID-19 pandemic (Wei et al., 2021, see Chapter 4 for details), frequent encounters of misinformation on social media may significantly shape people's beliefs and behavior about the COVID-19 pandemic. This is consistent with previous studies in terms of information sources about misinformation diffusion and consumption, indicating that verified users, especially institutions or organizations may play more prominent roles in the diffusion of misinformation consumed by the Chinese public (Chen et al.,

2020; Vraga & Bode, 2017). Moreover, the study also found a link between user gender and misinformation engagement—debunking posts were more likely to come from female users, while misinformation messages had a higher possibility from male users (Chen et al., 2020).

Finally, we found that a great number of the misinformation messages also included pictures and hashtags, which might increase the spreading of these messages. Nevertheless, the percentages were relatively low compared to debunking messages. In addition, misinformation messages were shorter and more likely to contain emotions and uncivil words than debunking messages.

To conclude, although we were unable to analyze COVID-19 misinformation data from all of our studied cities due to lack of access to big data from Facebook, Twitter, or Line, the findings based on Weibo data have several implications for policymakers in combating misinformation during a public crisis: (1) misinformation on popular social media channels appear to be more attractive (and thus more widely circulated) than other messages (e.g., debunking messages); (2) it is very difficult to reduce the proliferation of misinformation from the sources because, as the Weibo posts show, it comes from nowhere (no URLs to trace, and government and media sources account for a significant proportion of it). These two insights suggest that coping with misinformation on social media platforms is a big challenge to the government and public health authorities.

Building on these findings, next chapter will examine the dynamic process of the diffusion of misinformation about COVID-19 to uncover the patterns of the spread on social media platforms with a computational approach. From the user perspective, we will also investigate the vulnerability of receivers with different demographic characteristics who encounter misinformation in Chapter 4.

References

Allen, J., Arechar, A., Pennycook, G., & Rand, D. (2021). Scaling up fact-checking using the wisdom of crowds. *Science Advances, 7*(36), 1–10. https://doi.org/10.1126/sciadv.abf4393

Blei, D. M. (2012). Probabilistic topic models. *Communications of the ACM, 55*(4), 77–84. https://doi.org/10.1145/2133806.2133826

Chen, K., Chen, A., Zhang, J., Meng, J., & Shen, C. (2020). Conspiracy and debunking narratives about COVID-19 origins on Chinese social media: How it started and who is to blame. *Harvard Kennedy School (HKS) Misinformation Review, 1*(8), 1–30. https://doi.org/10.37016/mr-2020-50

Chen, X. (2022, May 5). At the moment of the new crown pneumonia epidemic, do not disturb. *Science and Technology Daily.* http://digitalpaper.stdaily.com/http_www.kjrb.com/kjrb/html/2022-05/05/content_534647.htm?div=-1

Garg, N., Schiebinger, L., Jurafsky, D., & Zou, J. (2018). Word embeddings quantify 100 years of gender and ethnic stereotypes. *Proceedings of the National Academy of Sciences, 115*(16), 3635–3644. https://doi.org/10.1073/pnas.1720347115

Grinberg, N., Joseph, K., Friedland, L., Swire-Thompson, B., & Lazer, D. (2019). Fake news on Twitter during the 2016 US presidential election. *Science, 363*(6425), 374–378. https://doi.org/10.1126/science.aau2706

Kim, H., & Tandoc, Jr., E. (2022). Consequences of online misinformation on COVID-19: Two potential pathways and disparity by eHealth literacy. *Frontiers in Psychology, 13*, 1–10. https://doi.org/10.3389/fpsyg.2022.783909

Kroon, A. C., Trilling, D., & Raats, T. (2021). Guilty by association: Using word embeddings to measure ethnic stereotypes in news coverage. *Journalism & Mass Communication Quarterly, 98*(2), 451–477. https://doi.org/10.1177/1077699020932304

Lazer, D. M. J., Baum, M. A., Benkler, Y., Berinsky, A. J., Greenhill, K. M., Menczer, F., … Zittrain, J. L. (2018). The science of fake news. *Science, 359*(6380), 1094–1096. https://doi.org/10.1126/science.aao2998

Liu, B. (2010). Sentiment analysis and subjectivity. *Handbook of Natural Language Processing, 2*, 627–666. https://doi.org/10.1201/9781420085938-c26

Nyhan, B., & Reifler, J. (2010). When corrections fail: The persistence of political misperceptions. *Political Behavior, 32*(2), 303–330. https://doi.org/10.1007/s11109-010-9112-2

Sina Weibo. (2021). *Weibo service user agreement.* https://weibo.com/signup/v5/protocol

Song, Y., Kwon, K. H., Xu, J., Huang, X., & Li, S. (2021). Curbing profanity online: A network-based diffusion analysis of profane speech on Chinese social media. *New Media & Society, 23*(5), 982–1003. https://doi.org/10.1177/1461444820905068

Southwell, B. G., Thorson, E. A., & Sheble, L. (2018). Introduction: Misinformation among mass audiences as a focus for inquiry. In B. G. Southwell, E. A. Thorson & L. Sheble (Eds.), *Misinformation and mass audiences* (pp. 1–12). University of Texas Press. https://doi.org/10.7560/314555-002

Tencent. (2022). *Tencent AI Lab Embedding Corpus for Chinese Words and Phrases: A corpus on continuous distributed representations of Chinese words and phrases.* https://ai.tencent.com/ailab/nlp/en/embedding.html

UNESCO. (2018). *Journalism, 'fake news' & disinformation: Handbook for journalism education and training.* Retrieved May 28, 2020, from https://unesdoc.unesco.org/ark:/48223/pf0000265552/PDF/265552eng.pdf.multi

Vosoughi, S., Roy, D., & Aral, S. (2018). The spread of true and false news online. *Science, 359*(6380), 1146–1151. https://doi.org/10.1126/science.aap9555

Vraga, E. K., & Bode, L. (2017). Using expert sources to correct health misinformation in social media. *Science Communication, 39*(5), 621–645. https://doi.org/10.1177/1075547017731776

Wei, L., Yao, E., & Zhang, H. (2021). Authoritarian responsiveness and political attitudes during COVID-19: Evidence from Weibo and a survey experiment. *Chinese Sociological Review*, 1–37. https://doi.org/10.1080/21620555.2021.1967737

Yang, K. C., Pierri, F., Hui, P. M., Axelrod, D., Torres-Lugo, C., Bryden, J., & Menczer, F. (2021). The Covid-19 infodemic: Twitter versus Facebook. *Big Data & Society, 8*(1), 1–16. https://doi.org/10.1177/20539517211013861

Zeng, J., & Chan, C.-H. (2021). A cross-national diagnosis of infodemics: Comparing the topical and temporal features of misinformation around COVID-19 in China, India, the US, Germany and France. *Online Information Review, 45*(4), 709–728. https://doi.org/10.1108/OIR-09-2020-0417

Zhang, L., Xu, L., & Zhang, W. (2017). Social media as amplification station: Factors that influence the speed of online public response to health emergencies. *Asian Journal of Communication, 27*(3), 322–338. https://doi.org/10.1080/01292986.2017.1290124

Zhou, X., & Zafarani, R. (2020). A survey of fake news: Fundamental theories, detection methods, and opportunities. *ACM Computing Surveys (CSUR), 53*(5), 1–40. https://doi.org/10.1145/3395046

3 Diffusion of Misinformation
Topological Characteristics and User Vulnerability

Sibo Wang and Hai Liang

Introduction

With the outbreaks of the COVID-19 pandemic, people's daily life has been restricted by a variety of anti-epidemic measures, such as lockdown, quarantine, and work-from-home, which has led to more screen time and more social networking. People also read, retweet, and discuss COVID-19-related news more often than any other topics, such as questions about all aspects of this epidemic, where it came from, how it transmits, what symptoms it has, where it's happening, and how should we respond among other things. An ocean of relevant information has emerged. Not only do public health authorities release on social media the latest policies and updates on the latest epidemic situation, but social media platforms also make it possible for ordinary users to post or publish content they create to discuss and spread related news and updates. As a result, a tsunami of COVID-19-themed "infodemic" has swept online social networks.

Since the outbreak of COVID-19 in late 2019, news about the disease has tended to receive very high attention, and thus it is easy to be a hot spot. Discussions of COVID-19 topics have become a gathering place for various kinds of intentionally or unintentionally fabricated misinformation about the disease. Some COVID-19 misinformation exaggerates the severity of the epidemic and creates a surge of anxiety and worries in the general public. Refer to Chapters 1 and 2 for specific examples of such misleading and inaccurate messages. As illustrated in Chapter 1, misinformation has brought different degrees of harm to people's well-being and health.

Stimulated by the large user base of social media and the convenience of sharing, resistance to the dissemination of this misinformation is unprecedentedly small. Exposed to a large amount of unsubstantiated information and the opinions of others, users are often affected and become contributors to the further diffusion of the information (Wang & Zhang, 2022; Zhou & Zafarani, 2019). Compared with the rigorous verification of the veracity of the information itself, the influence of the source publisher or disseminators of the information on social media is more likely to have an impact on the

DOI: 10.4324/9781003355984-3

judgment of users. A piece of widely disseminated misinformation may be released by a for-profit marketing account with a large fan base. Ordinary users can help spark it by making the news sound convincing and forward to others. In other cases, users who get no attention can use social bots to carry out the early diffusion and increase the credibility of the fake story.

The reason why a piece of true news from an ordinary user is widely disseminated may be that the source news is retweeted by an Internet influencer (i.e., Key Opinion Leader—aka KOL), which gives it more exposure, or it may also be that it tells a truth that readers are eager to know. This sort of diffusion path exactly reflects a unique feature of decentralized social media that is different from traditional news websites with a top-down propagation structure. In the above example, the profile information of users (the number of followers, verification status, the number of historical tweets, etc.) and different degrees of the scope of message transmission belong to propagation structure information. As the explicit embodiment of the different degrees of attractiveness finally brought about by the content and writing styles, it can complement the traditional misinformation detection based on textual feature modeling and become a powerful pillar for identifying misinformation.

Building on the previous chapter concerning the source and message characteristics of COVID-19 misinformation on Weibo, this chapter explores the distinguishable characteristics of misinformation in the propagation structure that are different from that of true information. To illustrate, suppose you are surfing social media and come across a widely retweeted message with a picture that says: "The Russian government has put 800 lions and tigers on the street to prevent people from gathering during the pandemic." Some questions will slide into your mind. It sounds ridiculous but is it true? Who posted this news? How do people react when they retweet? With a skeptical attitude, you will check the veracity of this post carefully and find the truth that Russia did not release any tigers and lions to combat the pandemic. The post has been accompanied by a picture of a film set in Johannesburg, South Africa, in 2016.

This example raises a set of new questions. How can such a piece of misinformation be reposted? Who is the super-spreader? What types of users are vulnerable to misinformation? Can researchers judge misinformation by modeling its existing propagation structure? Chapter 3 will address these major questions. In addition, using Weibo as a case study for the same reasons as Chapter 2 (e.g., lack of access to big data from Facebook or Twitter in Hong Kong, Singapore, and Taipei), we are interested in exploring the differences in these aspects between true and false information about COVID-19, as well as the differences in the topological characteristics of information dissemination on other topics during the same period compared with the epidemic topic.

In short, by constructing a dataset of true and false messages on Weibo during the pandemic, we pursue a comprehensive analysis of misinformation diffusion (intentionally or unintentionally, see Wang & Zhang, 2022), with a focus on the topological characteristics of the diffusion pattern, the profile information of participating users, and the textual features of the information content. Additionally, a machine learning classifier that can accurately identify the veracity of information about COVID-19 and generate the crucial propagation substructures is obtained by modeling the above aspects of features.

Modeling the Topological Structure of Misinformation: An Example

Problem Definition

We start with an equation to build the topological structure. $G = (V, E)$ is a directed graph representing an online social network, where V is the node set, including users on the social network, each node represents a social media user, and E is the edge set, including information transmission behavior on the social network, and each edge represents a repost or a comment. We use the cascade $c = (V_c, E_c)$ as the input of the model, which is a connected directed graph representing the whole propagation process of a piece of news n_c, where $Vc \subseteq V$ represents the set of all participants in the propagation process of news n_c in the social network G, f_u^{text} represents the textual feature vector of the post published by user u, f_u^p denotes the profile information features of user u, and $Ec \subseteq E$ denotes the set of edges passed during the propagation of news n_c.

We now illustrate this definition with an example: A piece of misinformation about Dr. Zhong Nanshan, a well-known Chinese anti-epidemic expert, published by a big V user (e.g., KOL) on Weibo with more than 650,000 followers on June 18, 2020. It claimed that Dr. Zhong flew to Beijing to help fight a new wave of epidemic outbreaks in Beijing. The post triggered 599 reposts and comments. A portion of the propagation behaviors in this cascade is shown in Figure 3.1.

The truth: This message used Zhong Nanshan's expired video, falsely claiming that he had parachuted into Beijing, although he was in Guangzhou at that time. Consequently, the blogger was deducted 10 credit scores for publishing misinformation and was banned for blogging for 15 days. In Figure 3.1, we draw each node in the cascade as a block to facilitate representing the characteristics of the node. The left side of each block lists the profile information of the author of the microblog, that is, f_u^p, including the number of his/her followers, the number of his/her followees (if user u follows user v, then u is the follower of v and v is the followee of u), his/her verification status, his/her verification reason, etc. On the right side is the original microblog.

To analyze the original text, we need to use natural language processing technology, by dividing sentences into words and performing the frequency

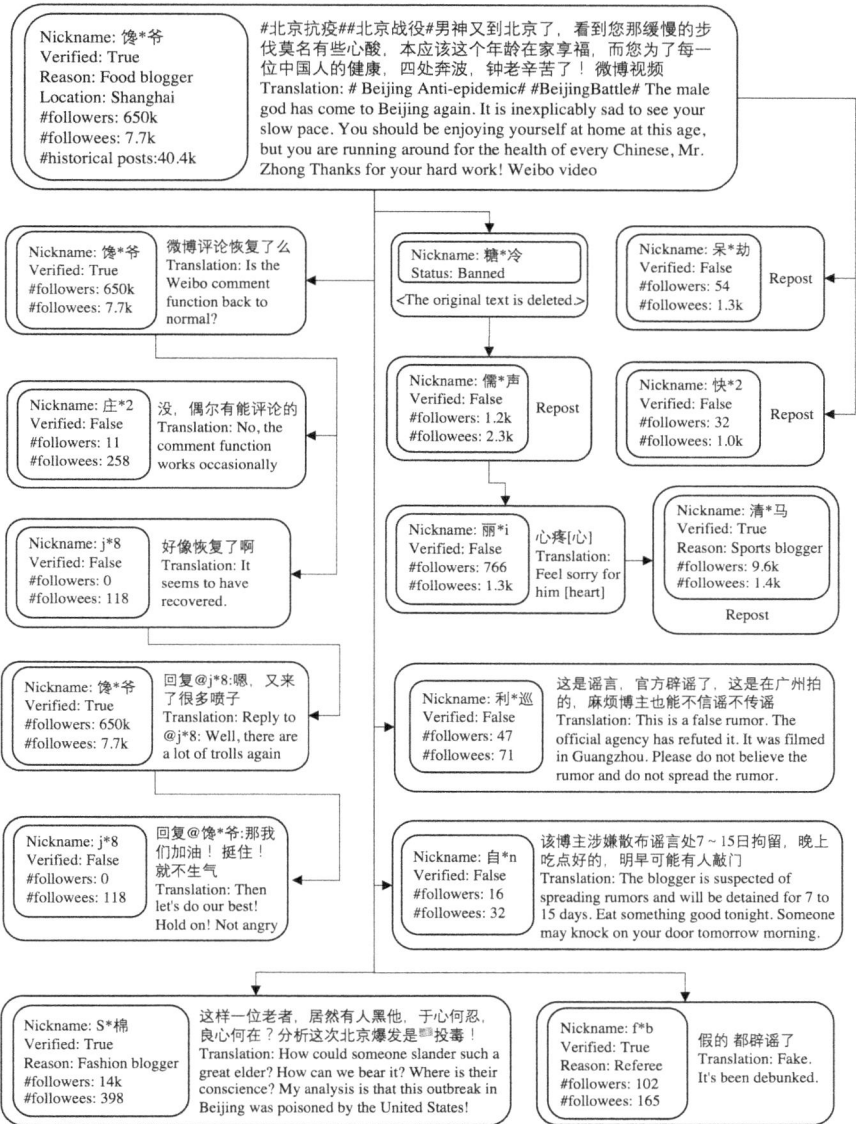

Figure 3.1 An example of cascade structure

statistics on the vocabulary, so as to constitute the textual feature of the microblog, namely f_u^{text}. The arrow in Figure 3.1 represents the edge we defined, that is, the flow of information, and the arrow pointing from node u to node v indicates that user v reposted or commented on the user u's post.

Topological Structure and Cascade Effect

By observing the substructure of the cascade drawn in Figure 3.1, we can get some statistics. For example, the maximum depth of the structure is 4, that is, the maximum length of the diffusion chain is 4, and the maximum breadth is 8, that is, a post is directly propagated at most eight times. All expressed in terms of concepts in graph theory, the node with the maximum outdegree has an outdegree of 8.

Similarly, we analyzed the complete cascade of the misinformation and visualized it in Figure 3.2, where each point represents the node of a microblog, and each arrow represents a directed information dissemination edge. The larger the area of a point, the greater the outdegree of the node. Users are also classified according to the user profile information represented by each node, and the detailed criteria will be explained later. The longest propagation path is also 4, and the node with the largest outdegree is the source post represented by the first block in Figure 3.1. The maximum outdegree is 568. That is, this microblog has been reposted and commented for 568 times, which is also the reason for the radial shape of the entire graph. Other than the source node, there are 20 nodes with outdegree greater than 0, indicating that 20 retweets generate information dissemination later. Using the two Chinese characters "谣" and "假" (rumor and fake) as keywords, we found that in the original cascade, 27 nodes questioned the authenticity of the source post like four microblogs at the bottom of Figure 3.1.

The above example illustrates that the introduction of topological structure in studying misinformation not only provides a perspective other than

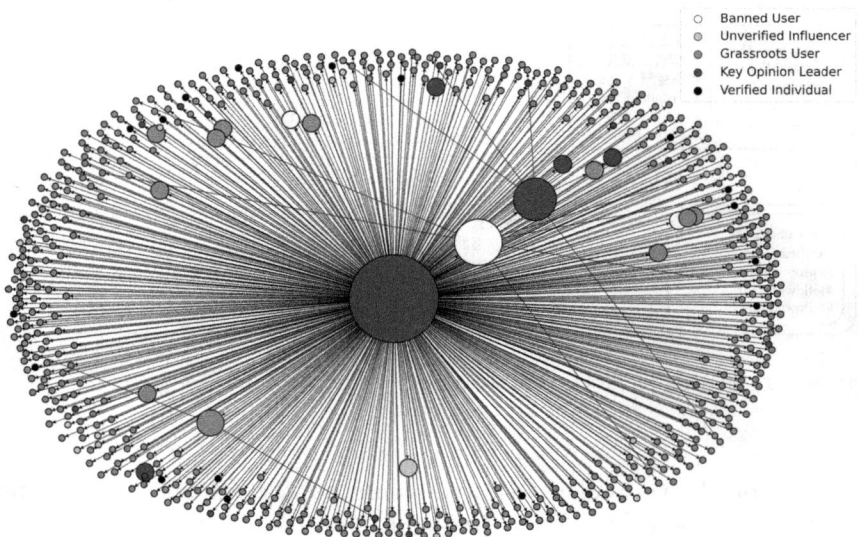

Figure 3.2 A complete cascade of misinformation diffusion

content to model it but also reveals more supplementary information in terms of text. We can capture evidence about the veracity of posts from different opinions about it expressed by all participants during its propagation. For the sake of comparison, we use true and false as the veracity expression of our two categories of information online, because fake news is more like a political metaphor.

Graph Structured Data and Analyses

Dataset

To study the characteristics of the topological structure of the misinformation related to COVID-19, we used Sina Weibo's API to collect and build a new dataset with a period from November 2019 to March 2022, including 4,174 source posts, which added up to 961,962 microblogs together with reposts from these sources. The user profile of the author of each microblog was also collected, including the number of followers, number of followees, verification status, verification type, verification reason, description, gender, location, etc. In addition, we scraped the number of historical posts by the users represented by root nodes. The misinformation came from Weibo Community Management Center (a service where users can report a microblog that contains false information), and social media posts collected according to COVID-19 misinformation on social networks published by China Internet Joint Rumor Suppression Platform. The true messages came from verifiably accurate items on official government accounts, the rumor-refuting microblogs provided by Weibo Community Management Center and microblogs posted by other users whose content and release time were consistent with the corresponding messages in the previous two sources.

Since we also sought to explore whether the dissemination characteristics of COVID-19 misinformation differed from those of other topics during the pandemic, this dataset included microblogs of other topics and their propagation cascades in the same period. We not only care whether there was a difference in the diffusion pattern of the true and false news of COVID-19 that could help us distinguish their veracity but also whether there was a difference between the spread of misinformation on COVID-19 and the spread of misinformation on other topics. Therefore, our dataset contained 2,171 cascades about COVID-19 and 2,003 cascades about other topics. In the same way, the misinformation came from Weibo Community Management Center, and the true information consisted of the corresponding rumor-refuting microblogs provided by Weibo Community Management Center and microblogs sampled from true messages collected according to Internet hot words during the pandemic. The details of the dataset are shown in Table 3.1, which is the largest Weibo dataset in the pandemic with comprehensive propagation structures of information.

Table 3.1 Details of the dataset built from Weibo

Dataset attribute	Weibo	Weibo-COVID-19 (COVID-19 subset)	Weibo-other (other topics subset)
#cascades	4,174	2,171	2,003
#microblogs	961,962	536,719	425,243
#microblogs per cascade	230	247	212
#cascades of true information	2,087	1,403	684
#cascades of false information	2,087	768	1,319
#microblogs in true cascades	650,600	484,152	166,448
#microblogs per true cascade	312	345	243
#microblogs in false cascades	311,362	52,567	258,795
#microblogs per false cascade	149	68	196

Analyses of Graph-Structured Data

According to the above statistical results in Table 3.1, the spread scope of true information was larger than that of false information, especially in the context of COVID-19. The size of cascades of true information was even five times that of false information, which leads us to regard topological structure as an important basis for judging misinformation. In addition, we also visualized the relationship between the amount of misinformation and the time span in the dataset by month. As Figure 3.3 shows, when COVID-19 was first known to the general public in January 2020, a sense of panic erupted on social media. Accompanied by the severity of the epidemic and the spread of cases, the amount of misinformation surged to a peak in March. This is consistent with the pattern in Chapter 2.

As the subsequent epidemic situation gradually came under control, misinformation rarely reappeared, although occasionally there was a small amount coinciding with a small rebound of the epidemic. Due to outbreaks of the highly contagious Omicron variant in China, the pandemic deteriorated sharply at the end of 2021, resulting in an amount of COVID-19 misinformation that reached a peak in January 2022. In other words, the emergence of COVID-19 misinformation on Weibo was closely related to the severity of the epidemic in China; when the epidemic was severe, the government generally adopted a strict lockdown policy, and it was difficult for the general public to rebut the misinformation on the spot, thus allowing rumormongers to send out misinformation. As Zhou and Zafarani (2019) pointed out, rumormongers tend to choose the time when people are most panicked, which further intensifies people's anxiety, makes them sensitive, and weakens their ability to discriminate the authenticity of the information, thus helping to spread misinformation.

Analyses of Diffusion Patterns

The characteristics of cascades of misinformation on Weibo in various aspects of its structural characteristics are shown in Table 3.2. Consistent with

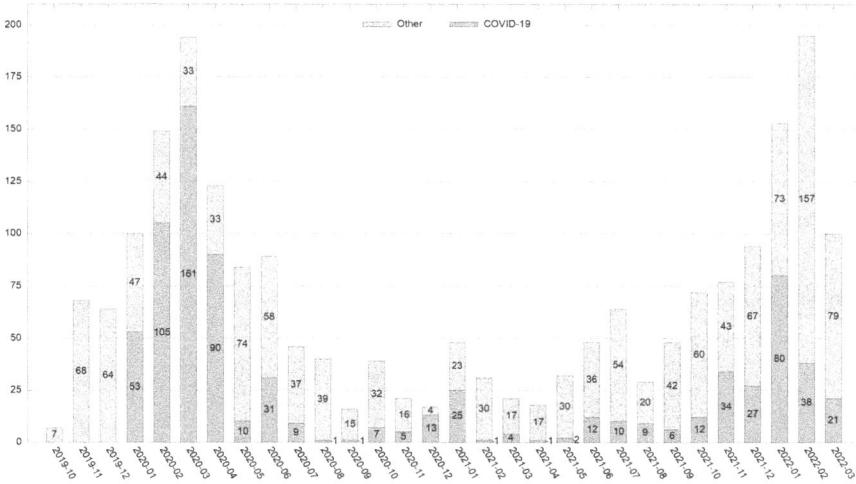

Figure 3.3 Misinformation over time

Table 3.1, in terms of the cascade size, the spread range of the misinformation was smaller than that of true news, but the dissemination of COVID-19 misinformation had been persistent following the initial outbreaks. For the longest path owned by a cascade, this metric also indicated the maximum depth of each cascade. The longest path of misinformation was longer than that of true information, suggesting that the spread of misinformation went deeper. That is, spreaders of misinformation were more likely to retweet comments of the source message than spreaders of true messages. The smallest standard deviation indicated that cascades of misinformation were the most stable in terms of maximum depth. In cascades, the nodes with the largest degree were generally the root nodes, and non-root nodes accounted for less than 4% of the four types of information.

Row "%Not root node" of attribute "Max Degree" in Table 3.2 represents the proportion of the most retweeted nodes that were not the root node in each category of information; it indicates that most of the super spreaders during the propagation process were the source post publishers, and only a small percentage of information spread more widely because it was reposted by others. On this metric, different from other topics, the probability that the node with the maximum degree of COVID-19 misinformation was not the root node was less than the true information. Statistics on the number of nodes with a degree greater than 1 in the cascade and their proportion in all nodes can reveal how many nodes further diffuse information. The proportion of nodes with further diffusion in misinformation was higher than that of true information.

Table 3.2 Structural characteristics statistics of COVID-19 misinformation on Weibo

	COVID-19 false	COVID-19 true	Other false	Other true
Cascade size				
Mean	68.45	345.08	196.21	243.35
Min	1	1	1	1
Median	6	4	11	9
Max	9,340	26,235	26,535	30,791
Longest path				
Mean	2.91	2.76	3.40	3.14
Std	1.95	1.97	2.59	2.41
Min	1	1	1	1
Median	2	2	3	2
Max	15	16	29	17
Max degree				
Mean	36.66	294.31	83.24	158.90
Min	0	0	0	0
Median	4	3	8	6
Max	2,640	22,063	7,805	22,348
%Not root node	3.65	3.99	3.26	2.78
Number of nodes with degree>1				
Mean	9.43	14.53	27.30	21.54
Min	0	0	0	0
Median	1	1	2	1
Max	1,363	1,210	3,705	1,954
Percentage	13.78%	4.21%	13.91%	8.85%

Who Is the Source?

In most cases, the authors of the microblogs represented by the root nodes of propagation cascades were the biggest spreaders in the entire propagation process. Specifically, we visualized the number of followers, followees, and historical posts of users of each cascade root node. For the sake of easy observation, we calculated the natural logarithm of these data and scaled the data to a certain range. As shown in Figure 3.4(a), the horizontal axis represents the number of followers, the vertical axis represents the number of followees, the area of each point represents the number of historical posts, and different markers of points represent different user verification statuses.

Message publishers of COVID-19 misinformation have an average of 340,989 followers, 1,314 followees, and 19,019 historical microblogs, while publishers of COVID-19 normal messages have an average of 16,941,965 followers, 1,109 followees, and 56,022 historical posts. According to the number of followers, it is clear that unverified users were mostly distributed in the left half of the figure, while verified users normally had larger orders of magnitude of followers. In contrast, misinformation has more unverified users in the right half of the figure (misinformation messages have more unverified

(a)

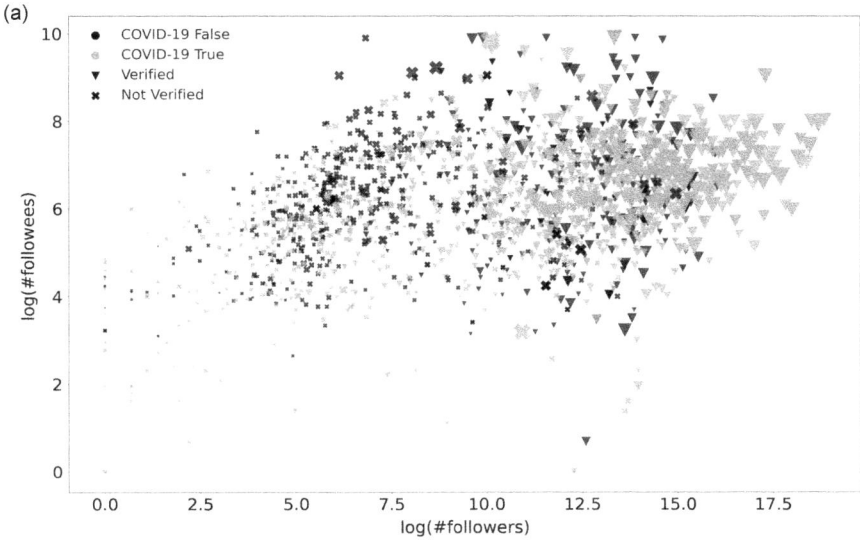

Figure 3.4(a) User profile information of source publishers where areas of points represent the number of historical posts

(b)

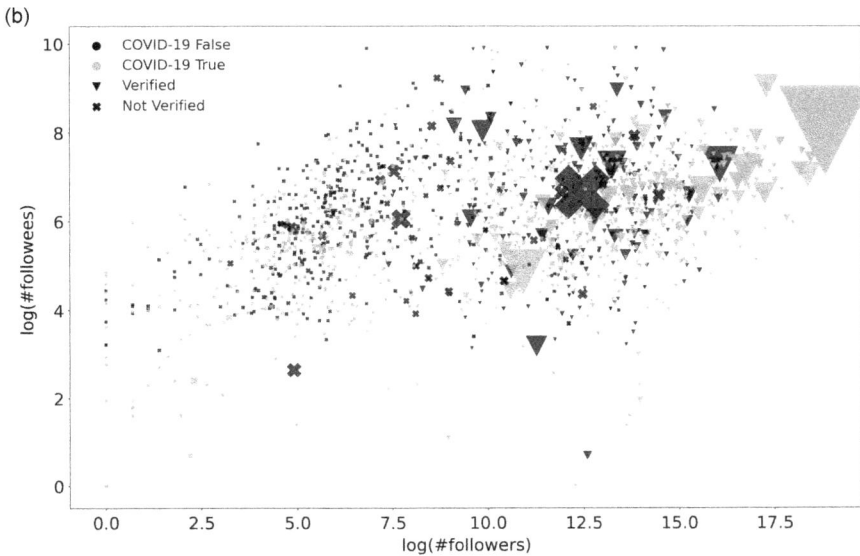

Figure 3.4(b) User profile information of source publishers where areas of points represent cascade size

publishers who have large fan bases than true messages), true information has more verified users in the left half of the graph (true messages own more verified publishers who have few followers than misinformation messages), and most of the publishers of true information are concentrated in the right half (most of the publishers of true messages have large fan base). With the increase in the order of magnitude of followers, the number of historical posts owned by users shows an overall upward trend, among which the average number of historical posts published by misinformation publishers is less than that of true information.

Do the source users during the propagation of COVID-19 misinformation have distinguishable geographical distribution characteristics? We carried out frequency statistics for the source users. On a scale from 1 to 100, Beijing (21.25%) was at the top of all provinces, followed by Guangdong (10.63%), Other (8.72%), Shanghai (8.17%), and Overseas (7.36%).

Further, we classified user nodes according to the number of followers, the number of followees, verification status, and account status. In line with the focus on diffusion patterns in this chapter, we took the dissemination potential reflected in each user's profile as a basis for classification, rather than the account type which has been analyzed in Chapter 2. To be specific, the sources with more followers can reach more users, while a microblog of a user with few followers had very low exposure. Consequently, we used the number of followers as one measure of transmission potential. The number of followees shows how widely a user receives posts from others. For example, a user who follows 2,000 accounts is more likely to see a particular message than someone who follows 100 accounts. Combining the two features, an account with a large number of followers but a much lower number of followees generally plays the role of an opinion leader on social media, such as *People's Daily* which has 150 million followers but only follows 3,000 accounts. Therefore, the ratio of the number of followers to the number of followees is also one of our dividing criteria. Besides, personal information is an important means to regulate users' behavior on the Internet for fear of being held accountable for inappropriate comments. The verification status, which requires the submission of real personal information to apply for, makes authors cautious in expressing their opinions and makes readers pay different attention to the judgment of microblogs posted by authors with different verification statuses. Similar to the processing method in Figure 3.4(a), we show the relationship between source user profile information and diffusion cascade size in Figure 3.4(b). It is clear that the area of the points near the upper right is larger, that is, messages posted by users with stronger influence potential are more widely spread. In addition, the points with a large area are generally verified users, indicating that messages disseminated widely, whether true or false, are more likely to be published by verified users.

In summary, the node type of the currently banned account is 0. For an unverified user, if the number of followers is greater than 500 and the number of followers is more than twice the number of followees, then node type 1, which represents users who tend to output opinions and have the potential to be influencers, namely unverified influencers, otherwise it is node type 2, which represents the grassroots users who tend to receive opinions; for a verified user, if the number of followers is greater than 10,000 and the number of followers is more than 20 times the number of followees, then the classification is node type 3, which represents the KOLs such as government accounts and Internet celebrities, otherwise, it is type 4, which represents the verified individual account. This classification method helps us to preliminarily divide users' influence potential on social media from the aspect of their profile information. Based on these user profile characteristics, we claim that type 3 users (KOLs) have the strongest influence potential, the weakest is type 2 (grassroots users), and type 0 (banned users) is not involved in the comparison as a specific category due to no accessible profile information. We visualized the distributions of user types under various conditions in Figure 3.5. Note that because some nodes included in a cascade may be from the same user, we used the user type of the author of each node to analyze the participation degree of this type during propagation, instead of only considering unique users. For instance, a cascade of misinformation contains ten tweets, but eight of them are from two grassroots users and only two are from two KOLs. Then the 1:1 result of these two user types can be calculated by the number of unique users, which misleads our judgment on the engagement of different types of users.

We then compared the node type distribution of publishers. As Figure 3.5 shows, except for COVID-19 misinformation, misinformation of other topics was mainly published by the most influential KOLs, while the users with the largest proportion of the publishers of COVID-19 misinformation were the least influential grassroots users. More than half of other kinds of information was posted by verified users, while COVID-19 misinformation was significantly smaller in the proportion of verified users. It is worth noting that when checking all the source user accounts in July, we found that 134 were already banned.

It is difficult to generalize about the main content of unverified users, but the verification reasons provided in verified accounts that make up the majority of sources can help us further understand COVID-19 misinformation rumormongers. We conducted keyword statistics on their verification reasons and found that We-Media was the majority, and their usual microblogs were related to star chasing, video, reading and writing, finance, science and technology, entertainment, etc. Except for medicine bloggers, there was little difference in the ability of bloggers in other fields to identify misinformation.

Who Is the Most Vulnerable?

Table 3.3 shows the proportions of node types of all tweets and unique users in the whole dataset, from which it is clear that grassroots dominated (79.23%) the category while KOL accounted for the least except for the

Table 3.3 Proportions of node types of all users in the dataset

Node type	0	1	2	3	4
User type	Banned users	Unverified influencers	Grassroots users	Key opinion leaders	Individual verified users
Tweets in the whole dataset					
Count	11,320	70,900	762,190	32,823	84,729
Percentage	1.18%	7.37%	79.23%	3.41%	8.81%
Unique users in Weibo-COVID-19					
Count	4,229	27,264	330,476	11,265	36,462
Percentage	1.03%	6.66%	80.66%	2.75%	8.90%
Unique users in Weibo-other					
Count	6,046	24,622	274,351	6,625	24,242
Percentage	1.80%	7.33%	81.68%	1.97%	7.22%

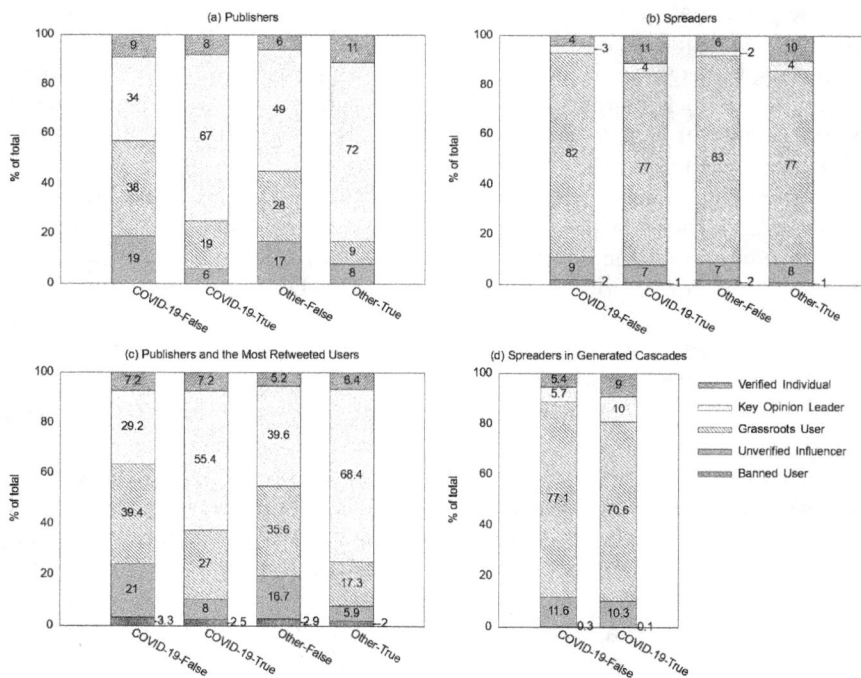

Figure 3.5 User type distributions under different conditions

banned users. This not only reveals that our dataset reasonably sampled the Weibo platform—where KOLs are a minority and grassroots users are the most common—but also reflects the different contributions of different types of users to the formation of the propagation cascades, which will be elaborated in combination with Figure 3.5.

For geographical distribution of all participants in COVID-19 misinformation propagation, Other (21.03%), Beijing (9.96%), Guangdong (9.74%), Shanghai (6.17%), and Overseas (5.53%) ranked in the top five regions on a scale from 1 to 100. The pattern shows the tendency of disseminators who hid their real identities.

According to Figure 3.5, grassroots users are indeed the most common type during the dissemination of information on social media, which occupies a dominant position regardless of the spread of true or false information. However, the proportion of grassroots users in the dissemination of misinformation is also significantly higher than that in true information. It can be concluded that the most common users on social media are the most vulnerable group and the main component of the dissemination structure of COVID-19 misinformation. The whopping 82% percentage of type 2 reveals that an overwhelming number of grassroots users participate in the cascade of misinformation dissemination. As the receivers of information, they can easily repost or comment on the microblogs they see, and the authenticity of the messages does not affect their information transmission behavior.

KOLs with the greatest influence represent the smallest proportion in the dissemination of each kind of information. As opinion leaders, they rarely participate in the further propagation of information but usually release the source microblogs as shown in Figure 3.5. Occupying second place in the misinformation dissemination user types are unverified influencers with greater influence among unverified users. Second place in true information dissemination goes to the less influential set of individual verified users. The proportion of verified users in the dissemination of misinformation is significantly smaller than that in the dissemination of true information. We can see how much influence can reflect how cautious users are about spreading behaviors. Verified users, as users with real-name information endorsements, generally have higher credibility and are more inclined to disseminate true information.

Table 3.2 shows that the root node was also the largest spreader in most cascades. Results obtained by directly counting the largest spreaders were the same as those shown in Figure 3.5. Therefore, we observed the node type distribution of both the root node and the largest spreader in the nodes other than the root node. Cascades smaller than 3 were excluded. As shown in Figure 3.5, grassroots users made the biggest contribution to the spread of COVID-19 misinformation; their proportion of 39.40% indicates that they were the super-spreaders of COVID misinformation. This is a very interesting phenomenon, because generally the microblogs that can be further spread are posted by users with enough fans or have rich textual characteristics, for example, they fully express personal views or are trolling. However, we note that most of the microblogs published by grassroots users contained only a few simple words. What causes such microblogs to get a lot of dissemination is worth further investigation.

At the same time, Figure 3.5 again reflects the opinion leader positioning of type 3 users. Although the proportion of KOLs decreased compared with the node type distribution of the root nodes in Figure 3.5, it still dominated the super-spreaders of the latter three kinds of information. Overall, there were more unverified users among the largest spreaders of misinformation, while there were more verified users among spreaders of real information. The largest spreaders in nodes other than the root node had a certain proportion of banned users, especially the highest proportion in COVID-19 misinformation. It should be noted that Weibo occasionally punishes misinformation spreaders by deducting credit scores. Banned users are usually a particular group of users whose statements involve sensitive topics and have a great impact, which are considered by Weibo authorities to have damaged the harmony of the online community. The proportion of type 0 shows the emergence of super spreaders who made comments that Weibo administrators considered very bad for hamony in the process of information transmission. For example, the account of Wang Sicong, one of the most famous rich second generation in China, was suspended after he published remarks that COVID-19 testing was actually a test of servility and questioned the effectiveness of Lianhua Qingwen Capsules.

To further explore the characteristics of COVID-19 misinformation diffusion patterns and user type distribution, we developed a Graph Convolutional Network model to combine and exploit the textual feature and topological structure of cascades in our Weibo-COVID-19 dataset, to predict the diffusion pattern and veracity, and finally achieve a good result of 93% accuracy in detecting misinformation task.

Our model simulated the crucial diffusion substructure by selecting a subset of important nodes in the complete propagation cascade. We visualized the node type distribution of all the participants in generated propagation patterns in Figure 3.5. Compared with the complete cascade shown in Figure 3.5, grassroots users remained the largest disseminator group, but the proportion decreased, while the proportion of verified users, especially KOLs, showed the largest improvement. When selecting nodes, our model tended to select nodes with more text information under the consideration of node features. As mentioned above, many grassroots users did not express their views on the source information, but just reposted microblogs. However, KOLs generally expressed their opinions on the source information, so the probability of being selected during training increased. The grassroots user base was large enough and consequently, there were enough text-informative candidates to choose from, so this only caused minor fluctuations in the proportions of the node types, which further confirmed that our model well captured the importance of different user types in determining cascade substructures whose information belongs to different categories.

Summary of Key Findings

Using big data from Weibo and computational methods and with a focus on identifying the topological characteristics of the diffusion pattern of COVID-19 misinformation as well as profiling Weibo users and the node types they represent, a number of patterns emerged in the present chapter. They shed light on how users propagate COVID-19 misinformation. Those patterns were compared with the dissemination of true messages. In summary,

- The emergence of COVID-19 misinformation on Weibo was closely related to the severity of the epidemic situation in China. With each outbreak, such as the early stage of the pandemic and the emergence of Omicron, the amount of misinformation soared to a peak. On the other hand, misinformation rarely appeared when the epidemic situation was under control.
- The spread range of COVID-19 misinformation was smaller than that of true messages, but the spread of misinformation went deeper (i.e., more disseminators of true messages retweeted the source microblog directly than that of misinformation).
- The sources concerning microblogs of COVID-19 misinformation spreading on Weibo were mostly published by KOLs and a large number of grassroots users; and they were mainly distributed in three of China's largest and most important cities: Beijing, Guangdong, and Shanghai. The largest proportion of misinformation sources were the least influential users (unverified with few followers).
- Most of the super-spreaders were the source post publishers, and the probability that the largest disseminator of COVID-19 misinformation was not the source publisher was less than that of true messages. The proportion of users who caused further retweets in misinformation was higher than that in true messages.
- Grassroots users were the most vulnerable group to COVID-19 misinformation. Using real-name and verification may reduce users' reposting unchecked misinformation messages on social media.

Conclusion and Insights

Leveraging the reposting function on Weibo, in this chapter, we tracked and reconstructed the complete diffusion paths of thousands of misinformation and normal messages. By doing so, we are able to identify the unique topological characteristics in the diffusion patterns of misinformation messages.

First, the source microblogs of COVID-19 misinformation spreading on Weibo were mostly published by KOLs and grassroots users and were mainly distributed in Beijing, Guangdong, and Shanghai. Consistent with a previous study (Goel et al., 2016), only a small proportion of messages spread widely and deeply through reposting. Most super-spreaders in the diffusion cascades were the source accounts, mainly including KOLs and grassroots users. This implies that policymakers should focus on the sources to cope with misinformation spreading. However, as we found in Chapter 2, it might be difficult to identify misinformation sources in advance because most do not include any external URLs and many of the accounts are government and media accounts. One possible way to solve the problem is to improve the misinformation literacy of local government and media account managers. In addition, it is also consistent with a previous study (Vosoughi et al., 2018) that misinformation messages generally spread deeper than do normal messages.

Second, given the importance of sources, we further analyzed their characteristics. The findings indicate that the largest proportion of misinformation sources are the least influential users (unverified with few followers). Given the sheer volume of these grassroots users, it might be difficult to identify them using automatic approaches.

Finally, our analyses also suggest that grassroots users are the most vulnerable group to COVID-19 misinformation. This is unsurprising because they are the majority of Weibo users. However, it demonstrates that purely focusing on the sources is insufficient to cope with misinformation. It might be equally important to improve the misinformation literacy of the general public. Our findings also indicate that using real-name and verification may reduce users' reposting misinformation messages.

Then, how does the diffused misinformation surrounding COVID-19 spread among the public? How much do people actually view and contribute to the spread by sharing? Also, in what ways do the exposure to and sharing of COVID-19 misinformation differ by social media users' demographics, social differentiators, and the city in which they live? Using large-scale survey data collected in the four studied cities, we examine these empirical questions in the next two chapters.

References

Goel, S., Anderson, A., Hofman, J., & Watts, D. J. (2016). The structural virality of online diffusion. *Management Science, 62*(1), 180–196. https://doi.org/10.1287/mnsc.2015.2158
Vosoughi, S., Roy, D., & Aral, S. (2018). The spread of true and false news online. *Science, 359*(6380), 1146–1151. http://doi.org/10.1126/science.aap9559
Wang, R., & Zhang, H. (2022). Who spread COVID-19 (mis)information online? Differential informedness, psychological mechanisms, and intervention strategies. *Computers in Human Behavior, 138*, 107486. https://doi.org/10.1016/j.chb.2022.107486
Zhou, X., & Zafarani, R. (2019). Network-based fake news detection: A pattern-driven approach. *ACM SIGKDD Explorations Newsletter, 21*(2), 48–60. https://doi.org/10.48550/arXiv.1906.04210

4 Exposure to Misinformation

Patterns and Predictors

Guanxiong Huang and Wenting Yu

Introduction

In the context of a global pandemic and infodemic, people tend to have a high level of uncertainty and fear of infection, motivating them to actively seek relevant information via various channels (Salvi et al., 2021). The proliferation of COVID-19 misinformation on social media has greatly increased their chance of encountering such misinformation. For example, over 20 million misleading posts related to COVID-19 have been detected and removed by Facebook and Instagram as of June 2021 (Wong, 2021). A survey in the United States showed that more than half of the respondents (57.60%) reported that they had been exposed to misinformation about COVID-19 vaccines (Lee et al., 2022). Similarly, exposure to misinformation was high in East and Southeast Asian societies, ranging from 20% to 60% of the adult populations (Chen et al., 2022; Luk et al., 2021; Soon & Goh, 2021). Thus, this chapter examines the demographic characteristics of citizens who are exposed to COVID-19 misinformation to delineate the patterns of exposure among the surveyed populations.

To be specific, this chapter presents the results of a systematic investigation of exposure to misinformation related to COVID-19 in Beijing, Hong Kong, Taipei, and Singapore. To be comprehensive, we examined misinformation exposure with two distinctive scales: general exposure to misinformation and exposure to specific messages with false claims. Exposure to specific messages with false claims is considered as a more objective measure and thus will be used consistently throughout the book; while the measure of general exposure to misinformation is used for this chapter only to enrich the findings. As discussed in Chapter 1, sociocultural contexts of the four culturally similar cities are different due to distinct political systems of each city and the level of access to digital information. To provide a holistic picture of the misinformation exposure patterns in the four societies we explore the individual-level factors underlying the patterns and situate these patterns in their broad social contexts.

DOI: 10.4324/9781003355984-4

Exposure to Misinformation in Four Asian Societies

As evidence presented in Chapter 1 has shown, misinformation about COVID-19 emerged in bursts and then spread broadly prior to peaking. Similar patterns are reported by others. For example, Luk and his colleagues (2021) examined the exposure among the Hong Kong adult population to a false statement that "smoking/alcohol drinking can protect against COVID-19." Through a phone survey, they found that about 20% of the respondents had been exposed to this claim. Moreover, they observed that it was related to a rise in tobacco and alcohol consumption during the pandemic (Luk et al., 2021). In Taiwan, a study using Google Trends data found that 39.30% of Taiwanese Googlers saw or read fake news from a digital media source during the pandemic (Chen et al., 2022). Similarly, 60% of people surveyed in Singapore reported viewing COVID-19 misinformation of some sort online (Soon & Goh, 2021).

Other studies have revealed how people's information-seeking behavior is altered by the proliferation of COVID-19 misinformation on social media outlets. Tandoc and Lee conducted a focus group study (2022) in which 89 Singaporean young adults expressed concerns about their parents receiving and sharing a lot of fake news via WhatsApp. Tandoc and Lee suggested that people adopted various information behaviors (e.g., information seeking, information scanning) to manage the uncertainty around the public health crisis and that their exposure to both true and false information shaped their protective behaviors. Kim et al. (2020) found that the more misinformation people were exposed to, the more likely they would engage in heuristic processing of, rather than thoughtfully digesting, the information. Their findings suggest that misinformation exposure may hinder the absorption and acceptance of correct, evidence-based information about a public health crisis.

Moreover, the antecedents of exposure to misinformation on social media platforms are diverse, ranging from individual-level variables, such as education level, media use (De Coninck et al., 2021), scientific knowledge, and political identity (Buchanan & Benson, 2019; Pennycook et al., 2018), to message factors, such as negative sentiments (Kumar et al., 2021).

For instance, a large-scale survey (De Coninck et al., 2021) of eight countries/regions including Hong Kong showed that information consumption from traditional media (i.e., newspapers, radio, television) decreased misinformation beliefs related to COVID-19, while digital media use promoted misinformation exposure and misbeliefs.

In addition, recent study (Lo et al., 2022) indicated the digital media environment as a key moderator of exposure to COVID-19 misinformation. A restrictive media environment that affords limited access to web-based information may motivate people to seek and consume more content online of all sorts, rendering them more vulnerable to exposure to misinformation than were people living in a free media environment. Using past research as our theoretical grounding, we examined the types of COVID-19 misinformation (e.g., infectiousness, transmission routes, protection measures, and vaccines) that our responders across the four societies encountered in social media platforms and tied the encounters to key demographic variables and predictors, both individual-level and societal-level.

Operationally, we examined COVID-19 misinformation exposure with two measures: general exposure and exposure to misinformation statements. We measured how often the 4,094 respondents that we surveyed were exposed to misinformation in two different ways: (1) general self-reported exposure and (2) exposure to specific popular yet undebunked false messages or posts about COVID-19 on social media platforms. The two measures complemented each other in gauging the level of encounters with misinformation.

First, for general exposure, respondents were asked how often they were exposed to four types of COVID-19 misinformation: (1) misinformation about the infectiousness of COVID-19, (2) misinformation about COVID-19 transmission channels, (3) misinformation about COVID-19 protection measures, and (4) misinformation about COVID-19 vaccines. The items were rated from 1 = "never" to 4 = "often." The mean score of these items formed the index of general exposure to COVID-19 misinformation (M = 1.82, SD = 0.78, α = .88).

Second, respondents were provided five messages with COVID-19 misinformation from Facebook, Twitter, or Weibo. The messages were selected from a pool of false messages or posts about COVID-19 that circulated online during the pandemic (see Introduction). The items were: (1) "mosquitoes can transmit COVID-19 virus"; (2) "5G mobile networks can transmit the COVID-19 virus"; (3) "drinking alcohol can kill COVID-19 virus"; (4) "Asians are more likely to be infected with COVID-19 virus than other races"; and (5) "non-inactivated COVID-19 vaccines will alter human DNA." A 4-point Likert scale was used to measure the frequency, where "1" meant never, and "4" meant often. Responses were averaged to create a combined measure of exposure to COVID-19 misinformation (M = 2.65, SD = 0.70, α = .88).

Findings

Patterns of Exposure to COVID-19 Misinformation

The general measure of exposure shows that more than half (60%) of the 4,094 respondents in the four Asian cities indicated they "sometimes" or "often" viewed each type of general misinformation about COVID-19. For each of the provided false messages, more than 20% of the respondents chose "sometimes" or "often." Among the five messages, the claim that "non-inactivated COVID-19 vaccines will alter human DNA" was viewed the most, i.e., by about one-third of the respondents (28.60%). These results are consistent with the literature, indicating that encountering widespread misinformation about COVID-19 was common and extensive across the four cities at the time of this study.

Gender and Exposure

We compared the exposure to COVID-19 misinformation between male and female respondents. Based on the t-test results (refer to Table 4.1a), some gender-based differences were found: male respondents ($M = 2.68$, $SD = 0.72$) were exposed to COVID-19 misinformation more frequently than were female respondents ($M = 2.62$, $SD = 0.68$), $t = 2.73$, $p < .01$. This pattern was consistent across all four types of general COVID-19 misinformation.

Compared to female respondents, male respondents were exposed to four out of the five misinformation statements more frequently. There was little gender difference in exposure to the statement "mosquitoes can transmit COVID-19 virus" ($t = -0.04$, $p > .05$), as 25.70% female and 26.30% male respondents had encountered it "sometimes" or "often." The comparison of the combined index, however, showed that male respondents ($M = 1.85$, $SD = 0.80$) were exposed to misinformation statements more frequently than were female respondents ($M = 1.78$, $SD = 0.76$), $t = 2.77$, $p < .01$ (refer to Table 4.1b).

Age and Exposure

To examine the difference between age and exposure to COVID-19 misinformation, we split the age of the respondents at the median to generate a group of younger (i.e., 18- to 39-year-old; $n = 2,051$) and a group of older respondents (i.e., 40- to 85-year-old; $n = 2,042$). Based on the results on t-tests, there was no significant difference between the younger and older respondents in general exposure to COVID-19 misinformation about its infectiousness, transmission routes, protection measures, and vaccine. The comparison of the combined index showed no statistical difference between younger and older adults ($t = -0.17$, $p > .05$).

Table 4.1a Gender differences in patterns of general exposure to COVID-19 misinformation

	Male (n = 1,978)	Female (n = 2,116)	
	M (SD)	M (SD)	t value
Exposure to misinformation about the infectiousness of COVID-19	2.67 (0.79)	2.61 (0.73)	2.23*
Exposure to misinformation about COVID-19 transmission routes	2.65 (0.85)	2.59 (0.80)	2.37*
Exposure to misinformation about COVID-19 protection measures	2.67 (0.86)	2.62 (0.83)	2.10*
Exposure to misinformation about COVID-19 vaccine	2.73 (0.87)	2.66 (0.84)	2.62**
Combined exposure index	2.68 (0.72)	2.62 (0.68)	2.73**

Note: The items were rated from 1 to 4, where 1 = never and 4 = often; M = mean, SD = standard deviations; **$p < .01$, *$p < .05$.

Table 4.1b Gender differences in patterns of exposure to COVID-19 misinformation messages

	Male (n = 1,978)	Female (n = 2,116)	
	M (SD)	M (SD)	t value
Mosquitoes can transmit COVID-19 virus	1.80 (0.93)	1.8 (0.91)	−0.04
5G mobile network can transmit COVID-19 virus	1.74 (0.97)	1.68 (0.94)	2.02*
Drinking alcohol can kill COVID-19 virus	1.87 (0.99)	1.77 (0.95)	3.31**
Non-inactivated COVID-19 vaccines will alter human DNA	1.94 (0.98)	1.88 (0.94)	2.19*
Asians are more likely to be infected with COVID-19 virus than others	1.89 (0.98)	1.78 (0.94)	3.76***
Combined exposure index	1.85 (0.80)	1.78 (0.76)	2.77**

Note: The items were rated from 1 to 4, where 1 = never and 4 = often; M = mean, SD = standard deviations; ***$p < .001$, **$p < .01$, *$p < .05$.

Table 4.2 Differences in patterns of exposure to COVID-19 misinformation messages between younger and older adults

	Younger adults (n = 2,051)	Older adults (n = 2,042)	
	M (SD)	M (SD)	t value
Mosquitoes can transmit COVID-19 virus	1.89 (0.943)	1.71 (0.89)	6.12***
5G mobile network can transmit COVID-19 virus	1.78 (0.99)	1.65 (0.92)	4.38***
Drinking alcohol can kill COVID-19 virus	1.87 (0.98)	1.76 (0.96)	3.67***
Non-inactivated COVID-19 vaccines will alter human DNA	1.96 (0.97)	1.86 (0.94)	3.07**
Asians are more likely to be infected with COVID-19 virus than others	1.89 (0.98)	1.78 (0.94)	3.95***
Combined exposure index	1.87 (0.79)	1.75 (0.77)	5.15***

Note: The items were rated from 1 to 4, where 1 = never and 4 = often; M = mean, SD = standard deviations; ***$p < .001$, **$p < .01$; the age entry has one missing value.

However, when it comes to exposure to specific misinformation statements, younger adults were exposed to each message more frequently than were older adults (refer to Table 4.2). The greatest difference was found in exposure to the claim that "mosquitoes can transmit COVID-19 virus." Among the 4,093 respondents, 29.30% of the younger adults were exposed to this statement "sometimes" or "often," while only 22.60% of the older adults were exposed to it "sometimes" or "often." The t-test results of the combined index between younger ($M = 1.87$, $SD = 0.79$) and older adults ($M = 1.75$, $SD = 0.77$) were significant ($t = 5.15$, $p < .001$).

Sharing and Exposure

Next, we explored whether exposure to COVID-19 misinformation was tied to the level of sharing of COVID-19 misinformation. Respondents were categorized into high-sharing (n = 1,757) and low-sharing (n = 2,337) groups (sharing was measured on a 4-point frequency scale (1 = never, 4 = often), M = 2.23, SD = 1.07). Results in Table 4.3a illustrate that compared to respondents who shared misinformation less (M = 2.52, SD = 0.72), respondents who shared misinformation more (M = 2.83, SD = 0.63) encountered misinformation more frequently (t = 14.55, p < .001). This happened probably because sharing makes the sender an active seeker of more of such information, resulting in greater exposure.

The pattern persisted when we examined exposure to the five misinformation statements (refer to Table 4.3b). Compared to respondents who shared misinformation less (M = 1.59, SD = 0.63), respondents who shared misinformation more (M = 2.11, SD = 0.86) were those who encountered misinformation more frequently (t = 21.65, p < .001). Indeed, exposure to COVID-19 misinformation varied by the amount of sharing with others. The more respondents shared the misinformation, the more they were exposed to it.

Perceived Interest of Others and Exposure

Exposure to COVID-19 misinformation also varied on respondents' perceived interest in misinformation of others. We classified the 4,094 respondents into three groups: those who perceived others as interested (n = 2,040), those who perceived others as neutral (n = 1,084), and those who perceived others as uninterested (n = 970). Significant differences across the three groups were found, $F(2, 4091)$ = 130.08, p < .001. Respondents who believed others to

Table 4.3a Differences in patterns of general exposure to COVID-19 misinformation between low-sharing people and high-sharing people

	High sharing (n = 1,757)	Low sharing (n = 2,337)	
	M (SD)	M (SD)	t value
Exposure to misinformation about the infectiousness of COVID-19	2.80 (0.71)	2.52 (0.77)	11.85***
Exposure to misinformation about COVID-19 transmission routes	2.83 (0.81)	2.46 (0.80)	14.70***
Exposure to misinformation about COVID-19 protection measures	2.83 (0.80)	2.51 (0.85)	12.40***
Exposure to misinformation about COVID-19 vaccine	2.85 (0.81)	2.58 (0.87)	10.06***
Combined exposure index	2.83 (0.63)	2.52 (0.72)	14.55***

Note: The items were rated from 1 to 4, where 1 = never and 4 = often; M = mean, SD = standard deviations; ***p < .001.

be interested in COVID-19 misinformation (M = 2.82, SD = 0.65) encountered each type of COVID-19 misinformation the most frequently, followed by respondents who perceived others as neutral (M = 2.52, SD = 0.67) and those who perceived others as uninterested (M = 2.44, SD = 0.75). These results suggest the role of "imagined others" in viewing misinformation about COVID-19 (Table 4.4a).

Table 4.3b Differences in patterns of exposure to COVID-19 misinformation messages between low-sharing people and high-sharing people

	High sharing (n = 1,757)	Low sharing (n = 2,337)	
	M (SD)	M (SD)	t value
Mosquitoes can transmit COVID-19 virus	2.13 (0.98)	1.56 (0.80)	20.21***
5G mobile network can transmit COVID-19 virus	2.03 (1.07)	1.47 (0.78)	18.53***
Drinking alcohol can kill COVID-19 virus	2.09 (1.05)	1.61 (0.85)	15.59***
Non-inactivated COVID-19 vaccines will alter human DNA	2.18 (1.02)	1.71 (0.86)	15.42***
Asians are more likely to be infected with COVID-19 virus than others	2.15 (1.03)	1.6 (0.83)	18.53***
Combined exposure index	2.11 (0.86)	1.59 (0.63)	21.65***

Note: The items were rated from 1 to 4, where 1 = never and 4 = often; M = mean, SD = standard deviations; ***p < .001.

Table 4.4a Differences in patterns of general exposure to COVID-19 misinformation along with the level of perceived interest of others

	Perceived others as interested (n = 2,040)	Perceived others as neutral (n = 1,084)	Perceived others as uninterested (n = 970)	
	M (SD)	M (SD)	M (SD)	F value
Exposure to misinformation about the infectiousness of COVID-19	2.81 (0.72)	2.52 (0.72)	2.42 (0.80)	111.43***
Exposure to misinformation about COVID-19 transmission routes	2.80 (0.82)	2.48 (0.76)	2.40 (0.82)	107.69***
Exposure to misinformation about COVID-19 protection measures	2.81 (0.83)	2.53 (0.78)	2.43 (0.87)	85.07***
Exposure to misinformation about COVID-19 vaccine	2.86 (0.83)	2.56 (0.81)	2.51 (0.89)	75.49***
Combined exposure index	2.82 (0.65)	2.52 (0.67)	2.44 (0.75)	130.08***

Note: The items were rated from 1 to 4, where 1 = never and 4 = often; M = mean, SD = standard deviations; ***p < .001.

Table 4.4b Differences in patterns of exposure to COVID-19 misinformation messages along with the level of perceived interest of others

	Interested (n = 2,040)	Neutral (n = 1,084)	Uninterested (n = 970)	
	M (SD)	M (SD)	M (SD)	F value
Mosquitoes can transmit COVID-19 virus	2.02 (0.98)	1.67 (0.83)	1.50 (0.76)	130.12***
5G mobile network can transmit COVID-19 virus	1.94 (1.06)	1.53 (0.78)	1.43 (0.77)	127.27***
Drinking alcohol can kill COVID-19 virus	2.02 (1.04)	1.65 (0.85)	1.59 (0.84)	90.69***
Non-inactivated COVID-19 vaccines will alter human DNA	2.10 (1.02)	1.77 (0.86)	1.65 (0.85)	91.05***
Asians are more likely to be infected with COVID-19 virus than others	2.05 (1.03)	1.67 (0.83)	1.57 (0.84)	107.63***
Combined exposure index	2.03 (0.85)	1.66 (0.65)	1.55 (0.63)	164.98***

Note: The items were rated from 1 to 4, where 1 = never and 4 = often; M = mean, SD = standard deviations; ***$p < .001$.

Table 4.4b showed that exposure to the five misinformation statements also differed on respondents' perceived interest of others, $F(2, 4091) = 164.98$, $p < .001$. Respondents who perceived others as interested in COVID-19 misinformation ($M = 2.03$, $SD = 0.85$) were exposed to the COVID-19 misinformation statements the most frequently, followed by respondents who perceived others as neutral ($M = 1.66$, $SD = 0.65$) and those who perceived others as uninterested ($M = 1.55$, $SD = 0.63$).

Together, the results indicate that those who thought others were interested in messages with claims that were half-true tended to view more of such messages.

Social Network Size and Exposure

We next analyzed whether the size of a respondent's social network played a role in affecting exposure to COVID-19 misinformation. Respondents were categorized into two groups based on their social network sizes on social media platforms such as Facebook and Instagram by a median split: large social-network group ($n = 2,099$) and small social-network group ($n = 1,995$). As results of t-test in Table 4.5a show, respondents with large social networks were exposed to each type of COVID-19 misinformation more frequently than those with small social networks, and the greatest difference lay in exposure to misinformation about COVID-19 transmission routes. There was a significant difference in the combined index of general exposure to COVID-19 misinformation ($t = 12.71$, $p < .001$) between respondents with large social networks ($M = 2.78$, $SD = 0.66$) and those with small social networks ($M = 2.51$, $SD = 0.71$).

Table 4.5a Differences in patterns of general exposure to COVID-19 misinformation between people with small social network size and people with large social network size

	Large social network size (n = 2,099)	Small social network size (n = 1,995)	
	M (SD)	M (SD)	t value
Exposure to misinformation about the infectiousness of COVID-19	2.76 (0.74)	2.52 (0.76)	10.06***
Exposure to misinformation about COVID-19 transmission routes	2.78 (0.82)	2.45 (0.80)	13.04***
Exposure to misinformation about COVID-19 protection measures	2.79 (0.83)	2.50 (0.83)	11.13***
Exposure to misinformation about COVID-19 vaccine	2.82 (0.83)	2.57 (0.86)	9.16***
Combined exposure index	2.78 (0.66)	2.51 (0.71)	12.72***

Note: The items were rated from 1 to 4, where 1 = never and 4 = often; M = mean, SD = standard deviations; ***$p < .001$.

Table 4.5b Differences in patterns of exposure to COVID-19 misinformation messages between people with small social network size and people with large social network size

	Large social network size (n = 2,099)	Small social network size (n = 1,995)	
	M (SD)	M (SD)	t value
Mosquitoes can transmit COVID-19 virus	2.06 (0.97)	1.53 (0.78)	19.41***
5G mobile network can transmit COVID-19 virus	1.97 (1.06)	1.43 (0.75)	18.96***
Drinking alcohol can kill COVID-19 virus	2.07 (1.04)	1.55 (0.82)	17.89***
Non-inactivated COVID-19 vaccines will alter human DNA	2.14 (1.01)	1.67 (0.84)	15.93***
Asians are more likely to be infected with COVID-19 virus than others	2.10 (1.03)	1.55 (0.80)	19.22***
Combined exposure index	2.07 (0.85)	1.55 (0.59)	22.79***

Note: The items were rated from 1 to 4, where 1 = never and 4 = often; M = mean, SD = standard deviations; ***$p < .001$.

Moreover, respondents with large social networks were exposed to each of the listed misinformation statements more frequently than were respondents with small social networks (refer to Table 4.5b). The comparison of the mean score showed that respondents with large social networks ($M = 2.07, SD = 0.85$) encountered the misinformation statements more frequently than did respondents with small social networks [($M = 1.55, SD = 0.59$), $t = 22.79, p < .001$].

Misinformation Beliefs and Exposure

Do levels of exposure to COVID-19 misinformation differ by belief in the misinformation? To address this question, we split the misinformation belief scale at the median and generated the high-belief (n = 2,066) and low-belief (n = 2,028) groups (refer to Chapter 8 for detailed measures of misbeliefs). For each type of misinformation, respondents with high-misinformation belief had more exposure than respondents with low misinformation beliefs (refer to Table 4.6a). On average, respondents with high misinformation beliefs were exposed to COVID-19 misinformation more frequently (t = 3.92, p < .001). The results suggest a significant difference in how much respondents accepted false claims about COVID-19 as true and depending on the exposure the falsehood.

The pattern remained the same for exposure to specific misinformation statements (refer to Table 4.6b). Respondents with high misinformation belief (M = 2.05, SD = 0.82) were exposed to the statements more frequently than were respondents with low misinformation belief [(M = 1.56, SD = 0.67), t = 19.90, p < .001].

Knowledge and Exposure

To investigate whether exposure to COVID-19 misinformation differed on levels of knowledge about the COVID-19 pandemic, we separated respondents into a high-knowledge (n = 2,210) group and a low-knowledge (n = 1,884) group based on the median of the COVID-19 knowledge scale (the scale was provided in Chapter 8), and compared their difference in exposure to misinformation. Interestingly, respondents with high knowledge encountered all types of misinformation more frequently. Based on the t-test results

Table 4.6a Differences in patterns of general exposure to COVID-19 misinformation between people with high misinformation beliefs and people with low misinformation beliefs

	High misinformation belief (n = 2,028)	Low misinformation belief (n = 2,066)	
	M (SD)	M (SD)	t value
Exposure to misinformation about the infectiousness of COVID-19	2.68 (0.74)	2.61 (0.77)	3.03**
Exposure to misinformation about COVID-19 transmission routes	2.68 (0.83)	2.56 (0.81)	4.81***
Exposure to misinformation about COVID-19 protection measures	2.69 (0.83)	2.60 (0.85)	3.47***
Exposure to misinformation about COVID-19 vaccine	2.73 (0.84)	2.67 (0.87)	2.11*
Combined exposure index	2.69 (0.67)	2.61 (0.72)	3.92***

Note: The items were rated from 1 to 4, where 1 = never and 4 = often; M = mean, SD = standard deviations; ***p < .001, **p < .01, *p < .05.

Table 4.6b Differences in patterns of exposure to COVID-19 misinformation messages between people with high misinformation beliefs and people with low misinformation beliefs

	High misinformation beliefs (n = 2,028)	Low misinformation beliefs (n = 2,066)	
	M (SD)	M (SD)	t value
Mosquitoes can transmit COVID-19 virus	2.97 (0.95)	1.54 (0.81)	18.92***
5G mobile network can transmit COVID-19 virus	1.95 (1.04)	1.48 (0.81)	16.19***
Drinking alcohol can kill COVID-19 virus	2.01 (1.01)	1.63 (0.89)	12.55***
Non-inactivated COVID-19 vaccines will alter human DNA	2.15 (0.98)	1.67 (0.87)	16.58***
Asians are more likely to be infected with COVID-19 virus than others	2.08 (1.00)	1.60 (0.87)	16.36***
Combined exposure index	2.05 (0.82)	1.56 (0.67)	19.90***

Note: The items were rated from 1 to 4, where 1 = never and 4 = often; M = mean, SD = standard deviations; ***p < .001.

Table 4.7a Differences in patterns of general exposure to COVID-19 misinformation between people with a high level of knowledge about COVID-19 and people with a low level of knowledge about COVID-19

	High knowledge (n = 2,210)	Low knowledge (n = 1,884)	
	M (SD)	M (SD)	t value
Exposure to misinformation about the infectiousness of COVID-19	2.70 (0.72)	2.57 (0.79)	5.26***
Exposure to misinformation about COVID-19 transmission routes	2.66 (0.80)	2.57 (0.85)	3.38**
Exposure to misinformation about COVID-19 protection measures	2.68 (0.81)	2.61 (0.88)	2.77**
Exposure to misinformation about COVID-19 vaccine	2.77 (0.83)	2.61 (0.87)	5.97***
Combined exposure index	2.70 (0.67)	2.59 (0.73)	5.07***

Note: The items were rated from 1 to 4, where 1 = never and 4 = often; M = mean, SD = standard deviations; ***p < .001, **p < .01.

of the combined index of general exposure, compared to respondents with low knowledge (M = 2.59, SD = 0.73), respondents with high knowledge (M = 2.70, SD = 0.67) had a higher level of general misinformation exposure (t = 5.07, p < .001) (refer to Table 4.7a). People of high knowledge tend to have stronger need for information, and active information-seeking can also lead to greater misinformation exposure.

Table 4.7b Differences in patterns of exposure to COVID-19 misinformation messages between people with a high level of knowledge about COVID-19 and people with a low level of knowledge about COVID-19

	High knowledge (n = 2,210)	Low knowledge (n = 1,884)	
	M (SD)	M (SD)	t value
Mosquitoes can transmit COVID-19 virus	1.66 (0.86)	1.96 (0.97)	–10.43***
5G mobile network can transmit COVID-19 virus	1.60 (0.89)	1.84 (1.01)	–7.70***
Drinking alcohol can kill COVID-19 virus	1.76 (0.93)	1.89 (1.01)	–4.50***
Non-inactivated COVID-19 vaccines will alter human DNA	1.86 (0.92)	1.97 (1.00)	–3.71***
Asians are more likely to be infected with COVID-19 virus than others	1.76 (0.91)	1.93 (1.01)	–5.61***
Combined exposure index	1.73 (0.71)	1.92 (0.85)	–7.71***

Note: The items were rated from 1 to 4, where 1 = never and 4 = often; M = mean, SD = standard deviations; ***$p < .001$.

However, when we compared the difference in exposure to misinformation statements, we found a reversed pattern (refer to Table 4.7b)—Respondents with high knowledge were exposed to the provided list of misinformation claims less frequently (*M* = 1.73, *SD* = 0.71), compared to the less knowledgeable respondents (*M* = 1.92, *SD* = 0.85), *t* = –7.71, *p* < .001. The different measures that we used may account for these inconsistent results. It is possible that people of high knowledge seek health information from more reliable sources, which reduces their chances of encountering misinformation that circulate widely on social media.

Cross-City Differences in Exposure

Finally, we examined the difference in exposure to COVID-19 misinformation among respondents in Beijing, Taipei, Singapore, and Hong Kong. As we outlined earlier (see Introduction), a structural difference across the four cities is access to digital information online. According to the measures we developed, digital accessibility is high in Hong Kong and Singapore and low in Beijing. Taipei falls in between.

For the general exposure to types of COVID-19 misinformation, respondents in Beijing had more exposure than respondents in the other cities in most situations (refer to Table 4.8a). The greatest difference was found in exposure to misinformation about COVID-19 protection measures. The majority of Beijing respondents (62.20%) encountered misinformation about COVID-19 protection measures "sometimes" or "often," while 61.20% of Taipei

Table 4.8a Differences in patterns of general exposure to COVID-19 misinformation in Beijing, Hong Kong, Taipei, and Singapore

	Beijing (n = 1,033)	Hong Kong (n = 1,017)	Taipei (n = 1,019)	Singapore (n = 1,025)	Total	F value
Exposure to misinformation about the infectiousness of COVID-19	2.70 (0.78)	2.53 (0.69)	2.67 (0.77)	2.66 (0.77)	2.64(0.76)	10.82***
Exposure to misinformation about COVID-19 transmission routes	2.70 (0.88)	2.55 (0.80)	2.63 (0.78)	2.61 (0.82)	2.62 (0.82)	6.27***
Exposure to misinformation about COVID-19 protection measures	2.73 (0.90)	2.52 (0.77)	2.71 (0.82)	2.62 (0.86)	2.65 (0.84)	13.34***
Exposure to misinformation about COVID-19 vaccine	2.70 (0.88)	2.58 (0.79)	2.78 (0.83)	2.73 (0.90)	2.70 (0.86)	9.45***
Combined exposure index	2.71 (0.71)	2.54 (0.64)	2.70 (0.70)	2.65 (0.73)	2.65 (0.70)	11.71***

Note: The items were rated from 1 to 4, where 1 = never and 4 = often; ***$p < .001$.

respondents, 57.70% of Singapore respondents, and 52.60% of Hong Kong respondents encountered it "sometimes" or "often." When comparing the combined index of general exposure to COVID-19 misinformation, respondents in Beijing encountered misinformation more frequently than respondents in the other three cities, $F(3, 4090) = 88.51$, $p < .001$, and respondents in the other three cities showed no statistical difference in misinformation exposure.

A similar pattern was found when we examined exposure to specific misinformation statements across the four cities (refer to Table 4.8b). Respondents in Taipei, Singapore, and Hong Kong were exposed to all types of misinformation statements less than were respondents in Beijing. The statistical test showed that respondents in Beijing encountered misinformation more frequently than did respondents in the other three cities, $F(3, 4,090) = 11.71$, $p < .001$. However, no statistical difference in misinformation exposure was found among respondents in the other three cities.

As we expected, these results indicate that restricted access to digital information was indeed counter-productive. Respondents in Beijing sought and

Table 4.8b Differences in patterns of COVID-19 misinformation exposure messages in Beijing, Hong Kong, Taipei, and Singapore

	Beijing (n = 1,033)	Hong Kong (n = 1,017)	Taipei (n = 1,019)	Singapore (n = 1,025)	Total	F value
Mosquitoes can transmit COVID-19 virus	2.22(0.96)	1.73(0.84)	1.60(0.84)	1.65(0.91)	1.80(0.92)	104.17***
5G mobile network can transmit COVID-19 virus	2.05(1.03)	1.67(0.89)	1.50(0.84)	1.62(0.97)	1.71(0.96)	67.27***
Drinking alcohol can kill COVID-19 virus	2.21(1.02)	1.61(0.85)	1.78(0.93)	1.68(0.95)	1.82(0.97)	85.39***
Non-inactivated COVID-19 vaccines will alter human DNA	2.12(0.99)	1.89(0.90)	1.78(0.92)	1.85(0.98)	1.91(0.96)	25.31***
Asians are more likely to be infected with COVID-19 virus than others	2.13(1.04)	1.71(0.87)	1.78(0.92)	1.71(0.95)	1.83(0.96)	47.29***
Combined exposure index	2.15(0.82)	1.72(0.68)	1.69(0.71)	1.70(0.81)	1.82(0.78)	88.51***

Note: The items were rated from 1 to 4, where 1 = never and 4 = often; ***$p < .001$.

consumed more content from online sources about the COVID-19 pandemic regardless of whether it were true, resulting in greater exposure to misinformation. On the other hand, respondents in cities with free access to web-based information viewed less of the misinformation because a full range of information about the pandemic was available. That is, free access to digital information actually reduced exposure to misinformation; whereas restricted access with blocks and firewalls led to increased exposure to such misinformation, a result consistent with the literature (Lo et al., 2022; Wei et al., 2022).

Predictors of Exposure

To go beyond bivariate analyses, we proposed a multiple regression model to predict the general exposure to COVID-19 misinformation with the following variables as predictors: key demographics, information accessibility (for measures, refer to Introduction), media use (e.g., frequency of consuming newspapers, TV news, online news and on social media), and social network size (e.g., the number of people in respondents' social media groups).

Based on the regression results shown in Table 4.9a, male respondents (β = .03, p < .05) who were more educated (β = .11, p < .001) were exposed to COVID-19 misinformation more frequently. Age was not a significant predictor of general exposure to misinformation (β = .01, p > .05). Respondents surveyed in cities with a higher level of information accessibility were exposed to general misinformation less frequently (β = −.05, p < .01). The use of newspapers (β = .17, p < .001), TV news (β = .07, p < .001), and social media news (β = .16, p < .001) were positively related to general exposure to misinformation, while use of online news (β = .03, p > .05) was not significantly related to general exposure to misinformation. In addition, social network size was found to be a positive predictor of general exposure to misinformation (β = .13, p < .001), which means respondents with larger social networks were exposed to misinformation more.

Similarly, we treated the combined index of exposure to misinformation statements as the dependent variable. We added general exposure to COVID-19 misinformation as a predictor in the regression model.

As Table 4.9b shows, male respondents were exposed to misinformation statements more frequently (β = .04, p < .05), while older

Table 4.9a Hierarchical regression analysis predicting the patterns of general exposure to misinformation

Predictors	General exposure to misinformation
Block 1: Demographics	
Gender (1 = Male)	.03*
Age	.01
Education	.11***
Adjusted R^2	2.3%
Block 2: Information accessibility	
Information accessibility	−.05**
Incremental adjusted R^2	0.3%
Block 3: Media use	
Newspapers	.17***
TV news	.07***
Online news	.03
Social media news	.16***
Incremental adjusted R^2	8.8%
Block 4: Social network size	
Social network size	.13***
Incremental adjusted R^2	1.5%
Total adjusted R^2	12.9%

Note: N = 4,093; ***p < .001, **p < .01, *p < .05; The age entry has one missing value.

respondents encountered the misinformation statements less frequently ($\beta = -.12$, $p < .001$). Education was not a significant predictor ($\beta = .01$, $p > .05$). Similar to the results in Table 4.9a, information accessibility was a negative predictor of exposure to misinformation statements ($\beta = -.18$, $p < .001$). Use of newspapers was positively related to exposure to misinformation statements ($\beta = .12$, $p < .001$), while use of TV news ($\beta = -.07$, $p < .001$) and online news ($\beta = -.15$, $p < .001$) were negatively related to the exposure. That is, respondents who accessed news from TV and the Internet more were exposed to the five popular misinformation statements less frequently. Social media news was not significantly related to exposure to the misinformation statements ($\beta = .02$, $p > .05$). Again, respondents with larger social networks were exposed to misinformation statements more frequently ($\beta = .19$, $p < .001$).

Additionally, general exposure to COVID-19 misinformation was a strong positive predictor of exposure to specific misinformation statements ($\beta = .34$, $p < .001$), indicating the more respondents encounter misinformation in general, the more they were exposed to specific false claims about the COVID-19 pandemic.

Table 4.9b Hierarchical regression analysis predicting the patterns of exposure to misinformation messages

Predictors	Exposure to misinformation statements
Block 1: Demographics	
Gender (1 = Male)	.04**
Age	−.12***
Education	.01
Adjusted R^2	1.5%
Block 2: Information accessibility	
Information accessibility	−.18***
Incremental adjusted R^2	4.1%
Block 3: Media use	
Newspapers	.12***
TV news	−.07***
Online news	−.15***
Social media news	.02
Incremental adjusted R^2	5.8%
Block 4: Social network size	
Social network size	.19***
Incremental adjusted R^2	5.0%
Block 5: General misinformation exposure	
General misinformation exposure	.34***
Incremental adjusted R^2	10.0%
Total adjusted R^2	26.4%

Note: N = 4,093; ***$p < .001$, **$p < .01$, *$p < .05$; The age entry has one missing value.

Summary of Key Findings

Findings in this chapter indicate that exposure to COVID-19 misinformation was prevalent among the four cities in our study. General patterns of misinformation exposure were found, including differences across the four cities.

- Male respondents encountered COVID-19 misinformation more frequently than did female respondents. Young adults were more frequently exposed to the COVID-19 misinformation statements than were older adults, but no significant age difference was found in exposure to general COVID-19 misinformation.
- Respondents who shared COVID-19 misinformation with others more frequently were exposed to COVID-19 misinformation more frequently. Similarly, respondents with high levels of misinformation belief also reported a higher frequency of exposure.
- The frequency of exposure to COVID-19 misinformation was highest among respondents who perceived others as interested in COVID-19 misinformation, followed by respondents who had neutral opinions and those who perceived others as not interested in COVID-19 misinformation.
- Respondents who had larger social networks on social media were exposed to COVID-19 misinformation more frequently than were those who had smaller social networks on social media.
- Respondents who were more knowledgeable about COVID-19 were exposed to misinformation more frequently than those who were less knowledgeable about COVID-19.
- Beijing, Taipei, and Singapore respondents were exposed to general COVID-19 misinformation more frequently than respondents in Hong Kong. When it comes to exposure to the specific COVID-19 misinformation messages, Beijing respondents reported a higher level of exposure than did respondents in Hong Kong, Taipei, and Singapore.
- Exposure to general COVID-19 misinformation was positively related to gender (male), education, social network size, traditional media use, and social media use, but it was negatively associated with the level of information accessibility. In terms of exposure to specific misinformation statements, gender (male), social network size, exposure to COVID-19 misinformation in general, traditional media use and Internet use were positive predictors, while age and the level of information accessibility were negative predictors.

Qualitative Findings

Encountering COVID-19 Misinformation

The focus group discussions confirmed that exposure to misinformation related to COVID-19 on social media was influenced by personal news consumption habit (i.e., news media use and interaction with social groups) and a macro-level factor (i.e., information accessibility). The discussions among the 80 participants revealed differences in news media use between younger and older adults. Young participants tended to obtain news from social media, including user-generated content. As Elijah, a 21-year-old Hong Kong student said, "I use the BBS LIHKG, where news about COVID-19 pops up automatically and I am exposed to it passively. I seldom seek more information through other channels." Theodore, a 26-year-old male sales rep working in Singapore said something along the same line. "I read news from Telegram, and also Facebook... I think it's also quite funny that I like to read all the comments." Noah, a 29-year-old male supermarket manager from Hong Kong, expressed his trust in social media as news source, "I like the KOLs and new media channels that I follow, and therefore I tend to believe what they post are true."

Although older adults also obtained news from online sources, they cared more about the credibility and quality of the sources, which might explain why they were exposed less to misinformation. Benjamin, a 58-year-old Hong Kong male accounting manager stated,

COVID information from the Hong Kong Department of Health is definitely reliable. Not sure about information from other sources. You can find a lot about COVID on YouTube, but you have to decide if it's trustworthy... We are facing too much information now. Sometimes if I hear something and I really want to know if it is true, I will go check the website of the Department of Health.

Similarly, Michael, a 40-year-old male game developer from Singapore, shared his experience:

I don't really use Facebook or other social media. I use more like Reddit and the WhatsApp group. So, I tried to avoid a group [echo] chamber because I think that if everyone in that group tends to be of a certain persuasion, and then it can tend to cascade on there. So, it's always good to have opposing views. And in the comment section, people will give different views and then I feel that I can make a more informed decision.

Participants also frequently encountered misinformation through online chats with people in their social groups. Amelia, a 39-year-old housewife from Hong Kong, described the misinformation she saw in WhatsApp as follows: "Usually I see the text with no source getting disseminated virally among WhatsApp groups. People just forward the text." Mr. Chang, a 33-year-old male flight attendant from Taiwan, received videos containing misinformation from his father. He recounted his story as follows: "My dad gets some false information from the video platforms. I think those messages are from mainland China. The popular COVID-19 misinformation is mostly about the prevention of coronavirus and the side effects of vaccines." Emma, a 33-year-old female and part-time yoga coach in Hong Kong, mentioned a specific piece of COVID-19 misinformation. "I have received a message," she recounted, "saying that drinking a mix of vinegar, lemon, and honey can improve immunity."

Ms. Zhu, a 41-year-old female in Beijing, recalled a message about COVID-19 vaccines that she received from friends.

> They said that the vaccine can stimulate cancer cells. Many cancer patients, no matter what kind of cancer they have, were told by doctors that the growth of cancer cells in their body is caused by the vaccine. They said that many doctors working in cancer hospitals said so... not only doctors in Beijing but also doctors from other regions.

Misinformation: "You Can Decide by Yourself"

Participants mentioned that they could tell sometimes that the information they encountered in online chats was not true, but they understood that their friends and family only shared the information with them out of a caring heart. As Emma, who received the anti-COVID recipe, explained, "People share the message with me through WhatsApp because they believe it's useful and want me to give it a try." Therefore, some participants said that they didn't mind reading the misinformation shared by friends and families. Abigail, a female fashion designer aged 37 from Singapore, described how she felt when she encountered misinformation:

> I actually welcome all the news that I receive on WhatsApp. I like to receive, and I like to listen or read it and I will decide whether to believe it or not. And I usually won't ask them to stop sending, stop circulating or tell them it's fake news. Because once they share, they somehow believe it. So, I don't think I'm in a position to like, discredit them from all this information they send because they care. So, I usually won't stop them unless they're my parents, then I will tell them it's a fake one. Other than that, I will just ignore after reading them... you can decide by yourself whether you want to listen or not.

Participants from the four cities recalled a great interest in COVID-19-related information at the early stage of the pandemic, when they actively looked for relevant information. Sophia, a 29-year-old female public servant in Hong Kong, said, "The government held press conferences to update COVID-19 cases at that time. And there was a post about it on BBS. So, like many others, I discussed with people online while watching the press conference." Jack, a 26-year-old male pricing analyst in Singapore, subscribed to news channels in Telegram to follow COVID-19 news. She explained, "I'm actually subscribed to CNA and Straits Times Telegram group. They have like a specific group for news. So, they have been quite handy. I always go to these channels when it comes to COVID-related news."

However, participants in cities of high information accessibility such as Singapore and Taipei tended to be skeptical about the information they received on social media. Mr. Kuo, a 27-year-old male paralegal in Taiwan said, "I feel suspicious about all the information I read. Any of them can be fake. You never know." However, participants in Beijing, a city of low level of information accessibility and a high level of pandemic control, were accustomed to learning about the latest information by hearsay or unofficial channels, even though they knew it could be wrong. Ms. Luo, a female sales manager aged 40, still remembered the time when there was a rumor about a possible lockdown in Beijing. Accord to her account, "When the rumor was spreading, my family immediately asked me to store up on things... It could be wrong, but people worried that they wouldn't get the time to buy groceries if the lockdown suddenly happened."

Ms. Zhu, also from Beijing, further explained the reason why she paid attention to the unverified information from social media platforms:

> If the neighborhood is closed down all of a sudden, you will be really nervous because you don't know what the actual situation is... We don't have a confirmed message from the authorities. There is no official word to tell us what is going on. In fact, it's not terrible to be locked inside; the major concern is that I don't know which part of the neighborhood is blocked and why. I don't know these things, so I am very anxious. All I can get is only some rumors heard from the neighbors.

Insights and Implications of Findings for Public Policy

The first conclusion we can draw from these findings is the common encounter of widespread misinformation on leading social media platforms in the four Asian cities (about 60%), which is on a par with similar studies in the United States (Lee et al., 2022). This particular finding shows that the infodemic is a global issue and Asia is no exception.

Based on the findings in the four cities, a profile of the respondents who are prone to encounter misinformation emerges: male, young, highly educated with a large social network on social media, and residents in a city with a low level of information accessibility. This finding meshes with numerous industry reports (e.g., CNNIC, 2022) that show netizens to be younger and better educated.

With regard to media use, the findings are consistent with previous studies in supporting the positive relationship between social media use and misinformation exposure (Chen et al., 2022; De Coninck et al., 2021). Our survey also suggests that traditional media use is positively related with misinformation exposure, while prior studies have indicated that traditional media use reduced misinformation beliefs (De Coninck et al., 2021). One possible explanation is that traditional media may serve as a source of debunking or fact-checking, which can mitigate the negative consequences of misinformation exposure. In Chapter 5, we further explore misbeliefs about COVID-19 as a result of exposure to the misinformation.

Finally, findings of this cross-societal study have implications for public policy in combating COVID-19 misinformation. Access and transparency are critical in shaping the encounter with such information. Firewalls and blocking that restrict access to digital information seem to be counter-productive. Thus, it is important for public health authorities and medical experts to have a presence on social media to engage in open and transparent communication with the public. In this way, whenever misinformation about COVID-19 or any other public health crisis appears on social media platforms, they can follow up with factual and evidence-based information to assist the public to fact-check user-generated content or to filter false information. In short, timely and accurate information presented by authoritative sources such as public health agencies should reduce the public's contact with misinformation that might gain popularity via sharing.

Apart from reducing misinformation circulated online to lower the chance of misinformation exposure, another perhaps more effective and sustainable way to combat misinformation during a public health crisis is to improve citizens' resilience to misinformation through timely debunking or correction practices and proper public literacy education programs.

Although respondents with the demographic characteristics described earlier may have higher chances of encountering misinformation during the COVID-19 pandemic, it does not mean they would necessarily be subject to the negative consequences of exposure to the misinformation. How does exposure relate to sharing the misinformation with others? What is the role of sharing together with exposure in leading to adverse effects of the misinformation? The next chapter—Sharing COVID-19 Misinformation—will examine these questions.

References

Buchanan, T., & Benson, V. (2019). Spreading disinformation on Facebook: Do trust in message source, risk propensity, or personality affect the organic reach of "fake news"? *Social Media + Society, 5*(4), 1–9. https://doi.org/10.1177/2056305119888654

Chen, Y. P., Chen, Y. Y., Yang, K. C., Lai, F., Huang, C. H., Chen, Y. N., & Tu, Y. C. (2022). The prevalence and impact of fake news on COVID-19 vaccination in Taiwan: Retrospective study of digital media. *Journal of Medical Internet Research, 24*(4), e36830. https://doi.org/10.2196/36830

China Internet Network Information Center (CNNIC). (2022). *The 49th Statistical Report on China's Internet Development.* Retrieved May 20, 2022, from https://www.cnnic.com.cn/IDR/ReportDownloads/202204/P020220424336135612575.pdf

De Coninck, D., Frissen, T., Matthijs, K., d'Haenens, L., Lits, G., Champagne-Poirier, O., ... Généreux, M. (2021). Beliefs in conspiracy theories and misinformation about COVID-19: Comparative perspectives on the role of anxiety, depression and exposure to and trust in information sources. *Frontiers in Psychology, 12*, 646394. https://doi.org/10.3389/fpsyg.2021.646394

Kim, H. K., Ahn, J., Atkinson, L., & Kahlor, L. A. (2020). Effects of COVID-19 misinformation on information seeking, avoidance, and processing: A multi-country comparative study. *Science Communication, 42*(5), 586–615. https://doi.org/10.1177/1075547020959670

Kumar, S., Huang, B., Cox, R. A. V., & Carley, K. M. (2021). An anatomical comparison of fake-news and trusted-news sharing pattern on Twitter. *Computational and Mathematical Organization Theory, 27*(2), 109–133. https://doi.org/10.1007/s10588-019-09305-5

Lee, S. K., Sun, J., Jang, S., & Connelly, S. (2022). Misinformation of COVID-19 vaccines and vaccine hesitancy. *Scientific Reports, 12*, 13681. https://doi.org/10.1038/s41598-022-17430-6

Lo, V., Wei, R., Lu, M., Zhang, X., & Qiu, J. L. (2022, May). *A comparative study of the impact of digital media environments, information processing and presumed influence on behavioral responses to COVID-19 misinformation in four Asian cities* [Paper presentation]. International Communication Association Annual Conference 2022, Paris, France.

Luk, T. T., Zhao, S., Weng, X., Wong, J. Y.-H., Wu, Y. S., Ho, S. Y., Lam, T. H., & Wang, M. P. (2021). Exposure to health misinformation about COVID-19 and increased tobacco and alcohol use: A population-based survey in Hong Kong. *Tobacco Control, 30*, 696–699. http://dx.doi.org/10.1136/tobaccocontrol-2020-055960

Pennycook, G., Cannon, T. D., & Rand, D. G. (2018). Prior exposure increases perceived accuracy of fake news. *Journal of Experimental Psychology: General, 147*(12), 1865–1880. https://doi.org/10.1037/xge0000465

Salvi, C., Iannello, P., Cancer, A., McClay, M., Rago, S., Dunsmoor, J. E., & Antonietti, A. (2021). Going viral: How fear, socio-cognitive polarization and problem-solving influence fake news detection and proliferation during COVID-19 pandemic. *Frontiers in Communication, 5*, 562588. https://doi.org/10.3389/fcomm.2020.562588

Soon, C., & Goh, S. (2021). Singaporeans' susceptibility to false information. *IPS Exchange Series No. 19*. https://lkyspp.nus.edu.sg/ips/publications?getCurrent=true&publicationtype=ips-exchange-series&year=&researchcenter=ips

Tandoc, Jr, E. C., & Lee, J. C. B. (2022). When viruses and misinformation spread: How young Singaporeans navigated uncertainty in the early stages of the COVID-19 outbreak. *New Media & Society, 24*(3), 778–796. https://doi.org/10.1177/1461444820968212

Wei, R., Guo, J., Wang, S., & Y.-H. C. Huang (2022). The role of digital information accessibility in shaping the relationships of exposure to COVID-19 misinformation and cognitive and attitudinal effects in Asia. *Communication and Society, 62*, 127–159.

Wong, Q. (2021, August 18). *Facebook removed more than 20 million posts for COVID-19 misinformation*. CNET. https://www.cnet.com/news/social-media/facebook-removed-more-than-20-million-posts-for-covid-19-misinformation/

5 Sharing Misinformation

Facilitating the Spread

Ven-Hwei Lo, Ran Wei, and Sai Wang

Introduction

Defined as the act of sharing content on digital media (Kümpel et al., 2015), sharing is a characteristic of social media communication. In fact, research shows that sharing of information and news on digital media has become the most popular means of acquiring or disseminating information (Purcell et al., 2010; Wei & Lo, 2021). Sharing extends the reach of a message to a large group of people. Sharing of information on social media can be done with the ease of a click or tap, including forwarding, redistributing the information by virtue of posting, reposting, retweeting, or recommending content with a "like" in addition to emailing.

What motivates people to share information online such as news? Previous research has identified a variety of motives such as socialization, information-seeking, status-seeking (Lee & Ma, 2012), self-expression (Chen et al., 2015), altruism (Apuke & Omar, 2021), and simply entertainment (Balakrishnan et al., 2021). Others have suggested that perceived issue importance, information utility, and ideological congruence also play a role in driving people to share news (Bobkowski, 2015; Su et al., 2019). As Goh et al. (2019) elaborated, people share news because sharing has social utility in generating mutual benefit between the sender and receiver.

Nevertheless, when it comes down to sharing user-generated content that includes unverified, false information, research has shown that even though sharing online represents a social good, if the shared information turns out to be false or misleading, sharing negatively impacts the sender's interpersonal relationships (Duffy et al., 2020; Hopp, 2022). Additionally, sharing fake news, even politically congruent fake news, can damage an individual's reputation in ways that are difficult to repair (Altay et al., 2022). Thus, if people can identify misinformation out of user-generated content, they are less likely to share it with others in their social circles. Under such a circumstance, Duffy et al. (2020, p. 1965) characterized the information as "too good not to share."

Putting the complicated relationship between exposure and sharing in the context of COVID-19 misinformation, we consider sharing of COVID-19

DOI: 10.4324/9781003355984-5

misinformation as the practice of social interactions by means of talking about, posting, or recommending to people in one's social circles information concerning the pandemic that is seemingly true but factually incorrect. Sharing represents a sort of post-exposure practice. As we presented in Chapter 4, a positive relationship exists between exposure to COVID-19 misinformation and sharing of it—the higher the level of exposure to the misinformation, the more frequently it is shared.

In addition, considering COVID-19 is an issue with high personal relevance and great social significance for a country's economy and citizens' well-being, others have suggested that people are likely to share COVID-19-related information regardless of whether true or false after exposure because they consider the information as important to themselves and others around them (Kim et al., 2020).

However, if the message is false, sharing it with others will lead to greater harm, such as confusing or misleading people who receive it. What is more, sharing with the purpose of convincing others that the information may be true may reinforce misbeliefs and make the information senders further ignore updated factual knowledge (Oyserman & Dawson, 2020).

In addition to trust in information shared via personal networks from sources with whom users have closer social ties (Yee, 2017), the social networks in which senders share misinformation also account for a great deal of the possible consequences—when misinformation is shared with people who lack sophisticated media literacy and Internet skills, sharing is likely to consolidate their false beliefs about COVID-19 and prevent them from learning scientific knowledge from media outlets. Therefore, it is important to seek a deeper understanding of sharing as a critical link in misinformation diffusion and acceptance.

Predictors of sharing of digital information on social media platforms are diverse, including demographics, cognition, and knowledge. For example, Chadwick and Vaccari (2019) found that males were more likely than females to share misinformation. Their findings also show the proportion of younger adults involved in misinformation sharing was higher than that of the elderly. Osmundsen et al. (2021) reported that people who were more knowledgeable about politics shared more fake news and misinformation. Accordingly, we anticipated that sharing of COVID-19 misinformation in the four cities would differ by individual-level variables, cognitive factors, and access to digital information at the societal level.

It is worth noting that sharing misinformation is a problem not confined to the West. The considerable number of connected populations in Asian countries seems to provide a fertile ground for spreading misleading information. The widespread use of social media and instant message apps (e.g., WeChat, WhatsApp, or LINE) in Asia enables people to exchange information, including unverified user-generated content, with others in their social circles. According to a recent report from the Statista Research Department (2021a), there were approximately 1.2 billion monthly active Facebook users in the Asia-Pacific region, making it one of the fastest-growing regions for Facebook users in the world (Williamson, 2020). As of December 2020, WeChat ranked first among the most popular Asia-based mobile messengers, with 1.23 billion monthly active users (Statista Research Department, 2021b). More notably, the daily average number of users on WeChat increased by 30% during the COVID-19 outbreak (WeChat Wiki, 2020).

Thus, we situate the process of COVID-19 misinformation diffusion through sharing in the broad context of the four societies in this chapter. Given the marked differences in access to digital information from social media platforms, we propose that in societies with higher information accessibility, where digital information is freely accessible and sharing can be socially beneficial, sharing COVID-19-related misinformation probably happens less frequently. Conversely, in societies with restricted information accessibility, misinformation sharing may occur more frequently, mainly because of the scarcity of diverse and authoritative information. In these circumstances, user-generated content fills the void of accurate and updated information about the pandemic. When this happens, information accessibility will likely result in more sharing of COVID-19 misinformation on leading social media platforms.

Our operationalization of sharing of COVID-19 misinformation relies on two measures: the frequency of sharing, i.e., how often respondents shared COVID-19 misinformation with people they know on social media on a 4-point scale (1 = never, 4 = often; M = 2.23, SD = 1.07); and the number of people shared (i.e., how many people with whom respondents shared COVID-19 misinformation).

Findings

Patterns of Sharing COVID-19 Misinformation

Simple frequency analysis of responses to the sharing questions showed that about one-third (28.90%) of the respondents acknowledged that they sometimes shared COVID-19 misinformation with others. About 14% indicated that they often engaged in sharing misinformation during the pandemic. One-third (34%) never shared COVID-19 misinformation with others. More than one-in-five (23%) respondents rarely shared such misinformation. In terms of number of people shared, among those (73%) who had shared misinformation with others, as many as 46.60% shared COVID-19 misinformation with 1–6 persons. About 16% of the respondents reported that they shared it with 7–12 persons, and 10% shared it with a dozen people or more.

Additionally, zero-order correlation between frequency and number of people shared was positive and strong (r = .59, p < .001), indicating the more often respondents shared the misinformation with others, the more people they shared with. Together, these results suggest that sharing false information about COVID-19 during the pandemic was common among the 4,094 respondents in the four cities, but the reach of the shared misinformation seemed to be limited, ranging from one to more than a dozen.

Age and Sharing

To explore whether the patterns of misinformation sharing differed across age groups, we split the age scale at the median to create two groups of younger (range = 18–39; *n* = 2,051) and older respondents (range = 40–85; *n* = 2,042). Among the younger respondents, nearly seven-tenths (69.70%) of them had shared COVID-19 misinformation. This tendency was slightly higher among older respondents (62.10%). As shown in Table 5.1, the difference in whether they had shared was significant, χ^2 (1, N = 4,093) = 27.78, *p* < .001, indicating that a greater proportion of younger respondents engaged in sharing COVID-19 misinformation than did older respondents.

As Table 5.2 further indicates, the results of an independent-samples *t*-test revealed a significant difference between younger respondents (*M* = 2.34, *SD* = 1.07) and older respondents (*M* = 2.12, *SD* = 1.05) in the frequency of COVID-19 misinformation sharing with others (*t* = 6.46, *p* < .001). Younger respondents consistently shared such misinformation more frequently than did older respondents.

However, regarding the number of people shared, there was no significant difference between younger respondents (*M* = 4.82, *SD* = 5.18) and older respondents (*M* = 4.63, *SD* = 5.64), *t* = 1.10, *p* > .05. Both groups shared

Table 5.1 Misinformation sharing across different groups

		Misinformation sharing		Chi-square value
		Yes	No	
Age	Younger respondents	69.74%	30.26%	27.78***
	Older respondents	62.14%	37.86%	
Gender	Male	66.13%	33.87%	.25
	Female	65.78%	34.22%	
Misinformation exposure	High level	71.85%	28.15%	47.96***
	Low level	60.91%	39.09%	
Perceived interest of others	Interested	83.87%	16.13%	728.26***
	Neutral	58.39%	41.61%	
	Uninterested	36.70%	63.30%	
Social network size	Large	77.99%	22.01%	236.94***
	Small	53.28%	46.72%	
Misinformation beliefs	High level	77.37%	22.63%	147.33***
	Low level	54.74%	45.26%	
Knowledge	High level	58.73%	41.27%	73.67***
	Low level	74.42%	25.58%	
City	Beijing	84.51%	15.49%	114.49***
	Hong Kong	73.75%	26.25%	
	Taipei	64.57%	35.43%	
	Singapore	69.07%	30.93%	

Note: ***p < .001.

COVID-19 misinformation with approximately 4.5 people in their social media circles. These results suggested that young people who were digital natives were more likely to engage in sharing COVID-19 misinformation on social media platforms. Older respondents, popularly known as digital immigrants, did not share as often as the digital natives.

Gender and Sharing

Based on the simple frequency analysis (see Table 5.1), the percentages of male respondents (66.10%) and female respondents (65.80%) who had shared COVID-19 misinformation with others were almost equal. Not surprisingly, the difference between gender and sharing COVID-19 misinformation was not statistically significant, χ^2 (1, N = 4,094) = 27.78, p > .05. As shown in Table 5.3, male respondents (M = 2.23, SD = 1.07) did not differ from female respondents (M = 2.23, SD = 1.06) in how often they shared the misinformation, either (t = .02, p > .05).

However, we found gender differences in the reach of misinformation sharing. Male respondents (n = 1,978) shared COVID-19 misinformation with more people than did female respondents (n = 2,116). On average, they shared with five people (SD = 5.71) on social media, whereas their female counterparts shared with nearly 4.5 people in average in their social network circles (SD = 5.11). Results of an independent-sample t-test indicated that the gender-based difference was significant (t = 3.56, p < .001) (Table 5.3).

Table 5.2 Differences in patterns of COVID-19 misinformation sharing between younger respondents and older respondents

	Older adults (n = 2,042)	Younger adults (n = 2,051)	t value
	M (SD)	M (SD)	
Frequency of sharing	2.12 (1.05)	2.34 (1.07)	6.46***
Number of people shared	4.63 (5.64)	4.82 (5.18)	1.10

Note: The scale for the frequency of sharing ranged from 1 to 4, where 1 = never and 4 = often. M = mean. SD = standard deviations. ***p < .001; The age entry has one missing value.

Table 5.3 Gender differences in patterns of COVID-19 misinformation sharing

	Male (n = 1,978)	Female (n = 2,116)	t value
	M (SD)	M (SD)	
Frequency of sharing	2.23 (1.07)	2.23 (1.06)	0.02
Number of people shared	5.04 (5.71)	4.43 (5.11)	3.56***

Note: The scale for the frequency of sharing ranged from 1 to 4, where 1 = never and 4 = often. M = mean. SD = standard deviations. ***p < .001.

Exposure to Misinformation and Sharing

To investigate whether exposure to COVID-19 misinformation was associated with the patterns of misinformation sharing, we distinguished high- and low-exposure respondents by splitting the exposure scale at the median (refer to Chapter 4 for the measurement). Nearly half of the 4,094 respondents were classified into the high-exposure group (n = 1,886) and the remainder into the low-exposure group (n = 2,208). As simple frequency analysis summarized in Table 5.1 shows, 71.90% of the high-exposure group had shared COVID-19 misinformation with others. The proportion of low-exposure respondents who had shared COVID-19 misinformation was lower at 60.90%. The difference between these two groups was significant, χ^2 (1, N = 4,094) = 47.96, p < .001.

The results of independent-samples t-tests show that high-exposure respondents (M = 2.45, SD = 1.11) shared misinformation more frequently with others than did low-exposure respondents (M = 2.04, SD = .99). That is, respondents who encountered misinformation more frequently were more likely to share misinformation with others. The difference between these two groups was also significant, t = 12.43, p < .001 (see Table 5.4).

Furthermore, high-exposure respondents (M = 5.96, SD = 5.99) shared misinformation with more people than did low-exposure respondents (M = 3.67, SD = 4.62). They shared misinformation with nearly six people, while the number of people the low-exposure group shared with was less than four. The difference between the two groups was significant as well (t = 13.54, p < .001). These results suggest that the more that respondents in the four cities were exposed to COVID-19 misinformation, the more frequently they shared it with others, and the more people they shared with.

Perceived Interest of Others and Sharing

The outbreaks of COVID-19 made people around the world worry about the global pandemic. Therefore, in addition to misinformation exposure, people might share COVID-19 misinformation with others because they

Table 5.4 Differences in patterns of COVID-19 misinformation sharing between low-exposure respondents and high-exposure respondents

	High exposure (n = 1,886)	Low exposure (n = 2,208)	t value
	M (SD)	M (SD)	
Frequency of sharing	2.45 (1.11)	2.04 (.99)	12.43***
Number of people shared	5.96 (5.99)	3.67 (4.62)	13.54***

Note: The scale for the frequency of sharing ranged from 1 to 4, where 1 = never and 4 = often. M = mean. SD = standard deviations. ***p < .001.

perceived that others within their social networks would want to hear about the disease. To explore whether the perceived interest of others was related to misinformation-sharing patterns, we differentiated the 4,094 respondents into three groups based on their answers to the question "In your opinion, how much are people within your social networks interested in the above-mentioned COVID-19 information that seems to be true but is actually false?" Respondents who indicated "Not interested at all" or "Not very interested" were categorized into the uninterested group (n = 2,040). Those who selected "Neutral" were classified into the neutral group (n = 1,084). Those who indicated "Somewhat interested" or "Very much interested" were categorized into the interested group (n = 970).

The results of simple frequency analysis show that the percentage of respondents who had shared COVID-19 misinformation with others was highest in the interested group (83.90%), followed by the neutral group (58.40%) and uninterested group (36.70%), χ^2 (2, N = 4,094) = 728.26, p < .001 (refer to Table 5.1).

As Table 5.5 shows, the frequency of sharing was highest among respondents who perceived others as interested in hearing about COVID-19 (M = 2.75, SD = 1.01), followed by people who had neutral opinions (M = 1.89, SD = .88) and those who perceived others as uninterested (M = 1.50, SD = .76). The differences between these three groups were statistically significant, $F(2, 4091)$ = 704.48, p < .001.

Further, a similar pattern was observed in the number of people shared. The number of people shared was largest among respondents who perceived others as interested in being informed about COVID-19 (M = 7.06, SD = 5.79), followed by respondents who had neutral opinions (M = 3.16, SD = 4.32) and those who perceived others as uninterested (M = 1.56, SD = 2.89). The number of interested people shared was twice as large as the neutral group, and six times as large as the uninterested group. The results of ANOVA tests show that these group-based differences were significant, $F(2, 4091)$ = 496.48, p < .001. It appears from these results that perceived interest of others in the information about COVID-19 was a motivator for sharing the misinformation online.

Table 5.5 Differences in patterns of COVID-19 misinformation sharing among interested, neutral, and uninterested groups

	Interested (n = 2,040)	Neutral (n = 1,084)	Uninterested (n = 970)	F value
	M (SD)	M (SD)	M (SD)	
Frequency of sharing	2.75 (1.01)	1.89 (.88)	1.50 (.76)	704.48***
Number of people shared	7.06 (5.79)	3.16 (4.32)	1.56 (2.89)	496.48***

Note: The scale for the frequency of sharing ranged from 1 to 4, where 1 = never and 4 = often. M = mean. SD = standard deviations. ***p < .001.

Social Network Size and Sharing

We further analyzed whether people with large social networks on social media (e.g., Facebook, Instagram) differed from people with small social networks in their misinformation-sharing behaviors. To do so, respondents were differentiated into small (n = 1,995) and large (n = 2,099) social network groups by splitting the scale at the median. Almost four-fifths (78%) of respondents with large social networks had shared COVID-19 misinformation with others. In comparison, the percentages of respondents with small social networks were lower, which accounted for 53.30%. The association between social network size and a respondent's sharing of misinformation was statistically significant, χ^2 (1, n = 4,094) = 236.94, p < .001(refer to Table 5.1).

According to results of independent-sample t-tests shown in Table 5.6, respondents with large social network (M = 2.57, SD = 1.06) reported a higher frequency of sharing COVID-19 misinformation than those with small social networks (M = 1.87, SD = .96), t = 22.13, p < .001. Moreover, a similar pattern was found for the number of people shared. That is, respondents with large social networks (M = 6.68, SD = 5.94) shared COVID-19 misinformation with more people than those with small networks (M = 2.66, SD = 3.84). The difference in the number of people shared was four (t = 25.81, p < .001). The patterns indicated that respondents who were active on social media with a large social circle tended to engage in sharing false information about the global pandemic.

Misinformation Beliefs and Sharing

To address whether misinformation beliefs were related to the patterns of misinformation sharing, we created two groups by splitting the misinformation belief scale at the median—high-belief (n = 2,028) and low-belief (n = 2,066) respondents (Chapter 8 has the details about the measure). It is unsurprising that nearly four-fifths (77.40%) of respondents with a high level of misinformation beliefs had shared COVID-19 misinformation with others. In comparison, the percentages of respondents with a low level of

Table 5.6 Differences in patterns of COVID-19 misinformation sharing between respondents with small social network size and respondents with large social network size

	Large social group (n = 2,099)	Small social group (n = 1,995)	t value
	M (SD)	M (SD)	
Frequency of sharing	2.57 (1.06)	1.87 (.96)	22.13***
Number of people shared	6.68 (5.94)	2.66 (3.84)	25.81***

Note: M = mean. SD = standard deviations. ***p < .001.

misinformation beliefs were lower at 54.70%. The association between respondents' misinformation beliefs and whether they had shared misinformation was statistically significant, χ^2 (1, n = 4,094) = 147.33, p < .001 (refer to Table 5.1).

As presented in Table 5.7, respondents with a higher level of misinformation beliefs (M = 2.48, SD = 1.02) shared misinformation more frequently with others than did those with a lower level of misinformation beliefs (M = 1.98, SD = 1.05). The results of independent-sample t-tests revealed that respondents with varying levels of misinformation beliefs differed in their COVID-19 misinformation sharing behaviors (t = 15.15, p < .001).

Moreover, a significant difference between these two groups in the number of people shared was found (t = 10.45, p < .001). Respondents with a higher level of misinformation beliefs (M = 5.60, SD = 5.49) shared misinformation with more people than did those with a lower level of misinformation beliefs (M = 3.86, SD = 5.20). Together, these results suggested that respondents who accepted false information about COVID-19 as true were more active in sharing such misinformation on social media platforms.

Knowledge of COVID-19 and Sharing

Would having knowledge about COVID-19 make a difference in sharing misinformation? To explore the question, we divided the knowledge scale at the mean to separate high-knowledge respondents (n = 2,210) from low-knowledge respondents (n = 1,884) (refer to Chapter 8 for measures used). As expected, nearly four-fifths (74.40%) of respondents in the low-knowledge group had shared COVID-19 misinformation with others. However, the proportion of high-knowledge respondents who had shared COVID-19 misinformation was much lower at 58.70%. The relationship between these two groups was statistically significant, χ^2 (1, N = 4,094) = 73.67, p < .001 (refer to Table 5.1).

As shown in Table 5.8, respondents who were more knowledgeable about COVID-19 (M = 2.05, SD = 1.05) shared misinformation less frequently than

Table 5.7 Differences in patterns of COVID-19 misinformation sharing between respondents with high misinformation beliefs and respondents with low misinformation beliefs

	High misinformation beliefs (n = 2,028)	Low misinformation beliefs (n = 2,066)	t value
	M (SD)	M (SD)	
Frequency of sharing	2.48 (1.02)	1.98 (1.05)	15.15***
Number of people shared	5.60 (5.49)	3.86 (5.20)	10.45***

Note: The scale for the frequency of sharing ranged from 1 to 4, where 1 = never and 4 = often. M = mean. SD = standard deviations. ***p < .001.

did those who were less knowledgeable about the disease (M = 2.43, SD = 1.05), t = 11.61, p < .001. Moreover, respondents who were more knowledgeable of COVID-19 (M = 4.21, SD = 5.28) shared misinformation with fewer people than did those who were less knowledgeable about COVID-19 (M = 5.32, SD = 5.52), t = 6.56, p < .001. Consistently, these results indicated that respondents who knew something about the COVID-19 pandemic shared less false and misleading information about it online.

Cross-City Differences in Sharing

As shown in Table 5.1, the results of the chi-square analysis of simple frequency indicated a significant difference in whether respondents in the four cities had shared COVID-19 misinformation with others, χ^2 (3, N = 4,094) = 114.49, p < .001. Specifically, the percentage of respondents who had shared misinformation was highest in Beijing (84.50%), followed by Hong Kong (73.80%), Singapore (69.10%), and Taipei (64.60%).

To further examine whether the mean difference in misinformation-sharing behaviors among four cities was significant, we conducted a series of ANOVA tests. As reported in Table 5.9, the results show that respondents from the four cities differed in the frequency of sharing COVID-19 misinformation, F(3, 4090) = 70.94, p < .001. The post-hoc Scheffe tests revealed that the Beijing respondents shared COVID-19 misinformation most frequently (M = 2.61, SD = 1.09), followed by the respondents in Hong Kong (M = 2.21, SD = 1.01) and Singapore (M = 2.11, SD = 1.01). Taipei respondents (M = 1.98, SD = 1.04) shared COVID-19 misinformation the least often. Additional post-hoc Scheffe tests show that these differences in the frequency of misinformation sharing among the respondents in the four cities were significant at the p < .05 level except for the difference between Singapore and Hong Kong respondents (p > .05).

In addition, there were significant differences between respondents in the four cities in the number of people with whom they shared the misinformation, F(3, 4090) = 85.27, p < .001. Specifically, the respondents in Beijing

Table 5.8 Differences in patterns of COVID-19 misinformation sharing between respondents with a high level of knowledge of COVID-19 and respondents with a low level of knowledge of COVID-19

	High knowledge (n = 2,210)	Low knowledge (n = 1,884)	t value
	M (SD)	M (SD)	
Frequency of sharing	2.05 (1.05)	2.43 (1.05)	11.61***
Number of people shared	4.21 (5.28)	5.32 (5.52)	6.56***

Note: The scale for the frequency of sharing ranged from 1 to 4, where 1 = never and 4 = often. M = mean. SD = standard deviations. ***p < .001.

Table 5.9 Cross-city differences in patterns of COVID-19 misinformation

	Beijing (n = 1,033)	Hong Kong (n = 1,017)	Taipei (n = 1,019)	Singapore (n = 1,025)	Total	F value
Frequency of sharing	2.61 (1.09)	2.21 (1.01)	1.98 (1.04)	2.11 (1.01)	2.23 (1.07)	70.94***
Number of people shared	6.95 (6.06)	4.34 (4.85)	3.82 (5.40)	3.75 (4.58)	4.72 (5.42)	85.27***

Note: The scale for the frequency of sharing ranged from 1 to 4, where 1 = never and 4 = often. Figures in parentheses are standard deviations. ***p < .001.

($M = 6.95$, $SD = 6.06$) shared COVID-19 misinformation with more people than did the respondents in Hong Kong ($M = 4.34$, $SD = 4.85$), Taipei ($M = 3.82$, $SD = 5.40$), and Singapore ($M = 3.75$, $SD = 4.58$). The post-hoc Scheffe tests indicated that the differences between Beijing respondents and respondents in the other three cities were significant at the p < .001 level. The number of people with whom Beijing respondents shared was seven, greater than Hong Kong, Taipei, and Singapore. However, there were no significant differences between Hong Kong and Singapore respondents (p > .05), between Taipei and Singapore respondents (p > .05), and between Taipei and Hong Kong respondents (p > .05).

Predictors of Sharing Behaviors

Finally, to examine which of the independent variables—demographics, information accessibility, exposure to COVID-19 misinformation, social network size, the perceived interest of others, misinformation beliefs, and knowledge of COVID-19—would have the most impact on misinformation-sharing behaviors, we first ran a series of correlation tests among the predictor variables and the sharing. Table 5.10 presents the correlation matrix, which indicates the zero-order relationships among all the studied variables were significant.

Based on the significant zero-order correlations, two separate hierarchical regression analyses were performed. As shown in Table 5.11 (column 1), gender was a significant but weak predictor of frequency of misinformation sharing ($\beta = .03$, p < .05), indicating that male respondents more frequently shared COVID-19 misinformation with others than did their female counterparts. Exposure to COVID-19 misinformation ($\beta = .13$, p < .001) was also significantly associated with the frequency of sharing misinformation. The results also show that the number of groups on social media was a significant and positive predictor ($\beta = .10$, p < .001); so were the cognitive variables such as perceived interest of others ($\beta = .45$, p < .001) and misinformation beliefs ($\beta = .11$, p < .001). Additionally, knowledge of COVID-19 was found to be a significant and negative predictor of misinformation-sharing frequency ($\beta = -.09$, p < .001), suggesting that having a good amount of knowledge of

Table 5.10 Bivariate correlations of key variables in the study

	1	2	3	4	5	6	7	8	9	10
1 Frequency of sharing	1									
2 Number of people shared	.59***	1								
3 Gender	0.00	-.54***	1							
4 Age	-.10***	-.02	-.17***	1						
5 Exposure to misinformation	.24***	.25***	-.04**	-.01	1					
6 Perceived interest of others	.55***	.49***	.04**	-.15***	.27***	1				
7 Social network size	.28***	.41***	-.01	-.02	.17***	.22***	1			
8 Misinformation beliefs	.33***	.27***	.01	-.03*	.15***	.22***	.26***	1		
9 Knowledge of COVID-19	-.18***	-.11***	-.16***	.12***	.11***	-.08***	-.11***	-.30***	1	
10 Information accessibility	-.15***	-.20***	.01	.04**	-.07***	-.20***	-.19***	.02	.03	1

***p < .001, **p < .01, *p < .05

COVID-19 could reduce the likelihood of sharing misinformation. Among these predictors, the perceived interest of others had the strongest effect on the frequency of misinformation sharing. Together, these predictors explained 37.70% of the variance in frequency of sharing COVID-19 misinformation.

With regard to the number of people shared with COVID-19 misinformation, regression analyses in Table 5.11 (column 2) found that both gender (β = .05, p < .001) and age (β = .05, p < .01) were significantly related to the number of people shared. Information accessibility (β = −.06, p < .001) and exposure to COVID-19 misinformation (β = .15, p < .001) also significantly predicted the number of people shared. Moreover, the number of social groups on social media (β = .25, p < .001), perceived interest of others (β = .38, p < .001), misinformation beliefs (β = .06, p < .001), and knowledge of COVID-19 (β = −.05, p < .05) were all significant predictors of the number of people shared. Consistently, perceived interest of others emerged as the strongest predictor of the number of people shared. The total variance accounted for by these significant predictors of number of people shared was 38.10%.

Table 5.11 Hierarchical regression analysis predicting the patterns of misinformation sharing

Predictors	Frequency of sharing	Number of people shared
Block 1: Demographics		
Gender (1 = Male)	.03*	.05***
Age	−.01	.05**
Education	.01	−.01
Adjusted R^2	1.0%	.03%
Block 2: Information accessibility		
Information accessibility	−.01	−.06***
Incremental adjusted R^2	2.1%	4.2%
Block 3: Exposure to COVID-19 misinformation		
Exposure to COVID-19 misinformation	.13***	.15***
Incremental adjusted R^2	11.3%	11.9%
Block 4: Social network size		
Social network size	.10***	.25***
Incremental adjusted R^2	3.0%	8.1%
Block 5: Perceived interest of others		
Perceived interest of others	.45***	.38***
Incremental adjusted R^2	18.3%	13.0%
Block 6: Misinformation beliefs		
Beliefs about COVID-19 misinformation	.11***	.06***
Incremental adjusted R^2	1.2%	0.4%
Block 7: Knowledge		
Knowledge of COVID-19	−.09***	−.05*
Incremental adjusted R^2	0.7%	0.2%
Total adjusted R^2	37.7%	38.1%

Note: N = 4,093; Beta weights are from final regression equation with all blocks of variables in the model. ***p < .001, **p < .01, *p < .05; The age entry has one missing value.

Summary of Key Findings

Findings of this chapter indicate that although misinformation sharing following exposure is a common phenomenon in the four surveyed cities, the patterns of sharing behavior tend to differ by the individual- and societal-level factors.

- More than half of respondents had shared COVID-19 misinformation with others. The number of people shared ranged from 1 to 6. Only a small number of respondents had shared misinformation with a dozen persons or more.
- Younger adults shared COVID-19 misinformation with others more frequently than did older adults. However, there was no significant difference between younger adults and older adults in terms of the number of people shared. Regarding gender, male respondents tended to share COVID-19 misinformation with more people than did female respondents. However, they did not differ in the frequency of sharing.
- Exposure to the misinformation about COVID-19 varies by the amount of sharing with others. The more respondents were exposed to misinformation, the more they shared; the more they shared, the greater exposure, suggesting a vicious cycle between exposure and sharing. In addition, high-level of exposure respondents not only shared misinformation with others more frequently but also shared misinformation with more people than did low-exposure respondents
- The more respondents perceived others as interested in COVID-19 misinformation, the more frequently they shared it, and the more people they shared with. In other words, sharing facilitated the spread of misinformation about the pandemic.
- Respondents with larger social networks on social media showed a higher frequency of sharing COVID-19 misinformation and a greater number of people shared than did those with small social networks.
- Compared to those with a lower level of misinformation beliefs, respondents with a higher level of misinformation beliefs not only shared misinformation more frequently but also shared misinformation with more people.
- The frequency of misinformation sharing, and the number of people shared were lower among respondents who were more knowledgeable about COVID-19.
- Respondents in Beijing shared COVID-19 misinformation most frequently, followed by the respondents in Hong Kong and Singapore. Taipei respondents shared COVID-19 misinformation least often. Moreover, the Beijing respondents shared COVID-19 misinformation with more people did than those in Hong Kong, Taipei, and Singapore.
- Factors that account for these differences in COVID-19 misinformation-sharing patterns include cognitive variables. Perceived interest of others

appears to be the strongest predictor of the frequency of sharing and the number of people shared. In addition, the number of social groups on social media plays a significant role in these two outcome variables. At the societal level, information accessibility is a negative predictor of misinformation sharing. It seems that people living in the city where they can easily access digital information of all sorts (e.g., Taipei) share misinformation with less people. By contrast, people living in a city with restricted information accessibility (e.g., Beijing) share misinformation with more people.

Qualitative Findings

Sharing or Not Sharing: A Hard Question

The remarks of focus group participants provided more nuanced insights into the reasoning behind sharing or not sharing misinformation surrounding COVID-19. Some people shared misinformation because they thought it was true. Michael, a 40-year-old male who worked for the IT industry in Singapore, cited the role of source credibility in misinformation sharing. In his words,

> People on Facebook. I'm sorry, but I have a very low view. I feel that Facebook is like the number one source of this information and because it's so easy to just share and then you can share passively, right. Let's say someone you really admire shares this post, then you say, oh, because this person shares this post, it must be true. And then you just don't verify and put in your WhatsApp group and then maybe your friends think if you are sharing this, this must be true and so on. And then that's how a lot of misinformation spreads.

Another cause of misinformation sharing is the lack of adequate knowledge about the virus. Camila, a 22-year-old student in Singapore, mentioned that in the early stage of the pandemic, she wanted to know as much as possible about the coronavirus. She recalled,

> At the start, we paid a lot of attention to any COVID news because we were very uneducated, we didn't know much about COVID. It's like the fear of the unknown. I just wanted to know anything they posted, such as the symptoms, the rules and everything because you wanted to educate yourself better.

She went on to say that she began to tune out information due to the fluctuating nature of the rules, particularly regarding the allowed size of social gatherings. "We always like to meet up with friends," she explained, "and I have a group of six, and then it's always a hard time making plans."

Due to lack of basic knowledge, participants frequently exchanged information with others on social media, including unverified information. Henry, a 51-year-old male working in the architectural industry in Hong Kong, mentioned a video about vaccination he received that he shared with others. He retold the story this way:

> I received a video… someone bled after vaccination, and the blood looked like glue. It was 2020 and not many people had taken the vaccines at that time. I shared it with others to see if they had encountered similar situations. After I got vaccinated, I knew more about vaccination, and then I stopped sharing it.

Participants also cited caring for others as a cause for sharing misinformation. Participants recalled that they often received misinformation from people around them. Gianna, a 31-year-old female in Singapore, said she received unverified information from her husband,

> My daughter got COVID when she was about 7–8 months old. And then I was so worried. My husband told me that babies won't die from COVID… they would get COVID but they won't die from it apparently because they're younger and their immune system is stronger. But I know there are so many babies who die from COVID.

True or Not, Just Share

Sophia, a 29-year-old female public servant in Hong Kong, told the group about her experience of sharing misinformation with her family. "I got a list of the restaurants that had COVID-19 infection cases in WhatsApp. I sent it to my family and told them to stay away from those places… But later I found out the information was fake." Similarly, Lucas, a 48-year-old male who works for finance in Hong Kong, shared with friends misinformation about a different matter. He remarked,

> Every once in a while, I received news in WeChat about mainland China reopening its border to Hong Kong… I actually knew the news was fake but I still forwarded it to friends who were eager to visit the mainland.

Avery, a 40-year-old female manager who works in the beauty industry in Singapore told a different story. She said that she had received some tips on being vaccinated from friends. Without consulting doctors or fact-checking the tips, she followed the advice, "My friends said before you go for the vaccination, you have to drink a lot of coconut water or tea and then drink a lot of water." Jack, a 26-year-old male pricing analyst in Singapore, acted differently for a different reason. Worried that his family could get fined by misinformation, he verified and shared the misinformation with a warning. He talked about a message saying that bleach could kill coronavirus,

> I think although it's a bit suspicious, I mean 80% of me doesn't believe it. But I think maybe my mom or my grandparents who are, you know, less misinformed, might actually believe it. So it becomes my responsibility to actually fact check that and let them know it is actually fake.

Participants in Beijing frequently mentioned that they shared messages, no matter true or not, to update family and friends. Due to the strict control policy in China. Ms. Zhao, a 36-year-old housewife living in Beijing, said as soon as she heard of COVID cases nearby, she shared it with people she knew. "I will ask everyone in the WeChat groups to be careful," she said. "We need to stay away from the places that have been hit with COVID cases. Also, if they have passed through those places, they need to do a quarantine at home or report it to authorities."

Other people just shared the messages about COVID for fun. Mr. Li, a 36-year-old male translator in Beijing, asked his friends about the reasons for sharing misinformation, such as drinking alcohol can kill the coronavirus. In his words, "They said they just shared it for fun. And their family won't take it seriously." Mr. Guo, a 43-year-old male who works in IT said, "We just share random things with each other. Sometimes you know the message is fake. We just see it as jokes."

Not Sharing After All

A few participants in our focus groups said they did not want to share misinformation because they thought it could hurt their reputation. Ella, a 27-year-old female who works in fintech in Singapore, called misinformation sharing a "scandal." She explained, "You get called out so easily on Tik Tok if you know you're spreading fake news. Then you create a whole scandal so yeah maybe not." William, a 49-year-old male engineer in Hong Kong, said something similar. According to him, "I don't always know if the message is true. If you share it with others, it may offend others." Liam, a 37-year-old male who is also an engineer from Hong Kong, worried that sharing misinformation might lead to bad consequences. "I discuss things with friends, face to face," he explained. "I don't discuss things on Facebook. People can start a fight with you there. You may even face the danger of being doxed."

Insights and Implications of Findings for Public Policy

Consistent with previous research (Chadwick & Vaccari, 2019; Seo et al., 2021; Wasserman et al., 2019), the findings of this chapter show that key demographics, such as age and gender, have been significant predictors of misinformation sharing during the global pandemic. Additionally, individual differences in exposure to COVID-19 misinformation, social network size, and the perceived interest of others also matter, suggesting a dynamic process of social interaction in the diffusion of the misinformation through sharing that involves individuals' social networks.

Importantly, beliefs of COVID-19 misinformation and knowledge about COVID-19 also affect the extent to which people share misinformation with others. It appears that the more the respondents are knowledgeable about the coronavirus, less they accept false claims in misinformation, and the less they shared COVID-19 misinformation. Such patterns underscore the power of knowledge in containing the spread of misinformation during a global pandemic. They also suggest that accepting falsehoods is a slippery road leading to widespread misinformation. However, having correct knowledge facilitates spreading correct knowledge about the pandemic. The implication for public policymakers in developing solutions to combat the spread of misinformation is to correct misinformation as soon as it is spotted. On the proactive side, health authorities need to educate the public about the pandemic with correct or fact-checked information. A well-educated public is critical to flattening the curve of the infodemic.

What's more, consistent with the results presented in Chapter 4, the role of societal differences in conditioning the sharing of misinformation by the respondents is demonstrated, leading to the generalization that the freer the information flow in a public health crisis, the less sharing of misinformation.

Taken together, these findings provide a comprehensive picture of various factors that have led to misinformation-sharing behaviors in the four cities studied during the global COVID-19 pandemic. What are the real-world consequences of exposure to the widespread of COVID-19 misinformation facilitated by sharing? In the following four chapters (e.g., Chapters 6–9), we will examine the influences of exposure and sharing of information about COVID-19 on respondents' negative emotions, risk perception, attitudes toward vaccines, misinformation beliefs, knowledge, and information overload.

References

Altay, S., Hacquin, A. S., & Mercier, H. (2022). Why do so few people share fake news? It hurts their reputation. *New Media & Society, 24*(6), 1303–1324. https://doi.org/10.1177/1461444820969893

Apuke, O. D., & Omar, B. (2021). Fake news and COVID-19: Modelling the predictors of fake news sharing among social media users. *Telematics and Informatics, 56*, 101475. https://doi.org/10.1016/j.tele.2020.101475

Balakrishnan, V., Ng, K. S., & Rahim, H. A. (2021). To share or not to share–The underlying motives of sharing fake news amidst the COVID-19 pandemic in Malaysia. *Technology in Society, 66*, 101676. https://doi.org/10.1016/j.techsoc.2021.101676

Bobkowski, P. S. (2015). Sharing the news: Effects of informational utility and opinion leadership on online news sharing. *Journalism & Mass Communication Quarterly, 92*(2), 320–345. https://doi.org/10.1177/1077699015573194

Chadwick, A., & Vaccari, C. (2019). *News sharing on UK social media: Misinformation, disinformation, and correction.* Online Civic Culture Centre, Loughborough University. https://repository.lboro.ac.uk/articles/report/News_sharing_on_UK_social_media_misinformation_disinformation_and_correction/9471269

Chen, X., Sin, S. C. J., Theng, Y. L., & Lee, C. S. (2015). Why students share misinformation on social media: Motivation, gender, and study-level differences. *The Journal of Academic Librarianship, 41*(5), 583–592. https://doi.org/10.1016/j.acalib.2015.07.003

Duffy, A., Tandoc, E., & Ling, R. (2020). Too good to be true, too good not to share: The social utility of fake news. *Information, Communication & Society, 23*(13), 1965–1979. https://doi.org/10.1080/1369118X.2019.1623904

Goh, D., Ling, R., Huang, L., & Liew, D. (2019). News sharing as reciprocal exchanges in social cohesion maintenance. *Information, Communication & Society, 22*(8), 1128–1144. https://doi.org/10.1080/1369118X.2017.1406973

Hopp, T. (2022). Fake news self-efficacy, fake news identification, and content sharing on Facebook. *Journal of Information Technology & Politics, 19*(2), 229–252. https://doi.org/10.1080/19331681.2021.1962778

Kim, J., Namkoong, K., & Chen, J. (2020). Predictors of online news-sharing intention in the US and South Korea: An application of the theory of reasoned action. *Communication Studies, 71*(2), 315–331. https://doi.org/10.1080/10510974.2020.1726427

Kümpel, A. S., Karnowski, V., & Keyling, T. (2015). News sharing in social media: A review of current research on news sharing users, content, and networks. *Social Media+ Society, 1*(2). https://doi.org/10.1177/2056305115610141

Lee, C. S., & Ma, L. (2012). News sharing in social media: The effect of gratifications and prior experience. *Computers in Human Behavior, 28*(2), 331–339. https://doi.org/10.1016/j.chb.2011.10.002

Osmundsen, M., Bor, A., Vahlstrup, P. B., Bechmann, A., & Petersen, M. B. (2021). Partisan polarization is the primary psychological motivation behind political fake news sharing on Twitter. *American Political Science Review*, 1–17. https://doi.org/10.1017/s0003055421000029028

Oyserman, D., & Dawson, A. (2020). Your fake news, our facts: Identity-based motivation shapes what we believe, share, and accept. In R. Greifeneder, M. Jaffe, E. Newman, & N. Schwarz (Eds.), *The psychology of fake news: Accepting, sharing, and correcting misinformation* (pp. 173–195). Routledge.

Purcell, K., Rainie, L., Mitchell, A., Rosenstiel, T., & Olmstead, K. (2010). Understanding the participatory news consumer. *Pew Internet and American Life Project, 1*, 19–21. https://assets.pewresearch.org/wpcontent/uploads/sites/13/legacy/Participatory_News_Consumer.pdf

Seo, H., Blomberg, M., Altschwager, D., & Vu, H. T. (2021). Vulnerable populations and misinformation: A mixed-methods approach to underserved older adults' online information assessment. *New Media & Society, 23*(7), 2012–2033. https://doi.org/10.1177/1461444820925041

Statista Research Department. (2021a, May 27). *Number of monthly active Facebook users in Asia Pacific from 1st quarter 2014 to 4th quarter 2020.* Statista. https://www.statista.com/statistics/652133/facebook-asia-pacific-mau-by-quarter/

Statista Research Department. (2021b, April 7). *Most popular Asia-based mobile messenger apps as of 4th quarter 2020, by number of monthly active users.* Statista. https://www.statista.com/statistics/250548/most-popular-asian-mobile-messengerapps/

Su, M. H., Liu, J., & McLeod, D. M. (2019). Pathways to news sharing: Issue frame perceptions and the likelihood of sharing. *Computers in Human Behavior, 91*, 201–210. https://doi.org/10.1016/j.chb.2018.09.026

Wasserman, H., Madrid-Morales, D., Mare, A., Ndlovu, K., Tully, M., Emejei, E., & Chikezie, E. U. (2019). Audience motivations for sharing dis-and misinformation: A comparative study in five sub-Saharan African countries. *Comparative Disinformation Workshop*. Harvard University. https://cyber.harvard.edu/sites/default/files/2019-12/%20Audience%20Motivations%20for%20Sharing%20Dis-%20and%20Misinformation.pdf

WeChat Wiki. (2020, August 3). *WeChat data, insights and statistics: User profile, behaviours, usages, market trends*. https://wechatwiki.com/wechat-resources/wechat-data-insighttrend-statistics/

Wei, R., & Lo, V. H. (2021). *News in their pockets: A cross-city comparative study of mobile news consumption in Asia*. Oxford University Press. https://doi.org/10.1093/oso/9780197523728.001.0001

Williamson, D. A. (2020, December 8). Global Facebook users 2020: The pandemic brought back momentum in lagging regions and led to even higher growth in others. *Insider Intelligence*. https://www.emarketer.com/content/global-facebook-users-2020

Yee, A. (2017). Post-truth politics & fake news in Asia. *Global Asia, 12*(2), 66–71. https://www.globalasia.org/v12no2/feature/post-truth-politics-and-fake-news-in-asia_andy-yee

6 Consequences of Exposure to Misinformation

Negative Emotions and Biased Risk Perception

Ven-Hwei Lo, Grace Xiao Zhang, and Miao Lu

Introduction

As discussed in Chapter 1, misinformation surrounding the COVID-19 pandemic is considered harmful to citizens around the world because it presents false and misleading claims that may misdirect people from accessing timely, accurate, and scientific information during the public health crisis (Ridder, 2021). Moreover, misinformation elicits a range of negative emotions about the pandemic, reducing people's subjective well-being (Pfefferbaum & North, 2020), and causing irrational behaviors such as panic buying (Zhang et al., 2020). In the early stage of the COVID-19 outbreak, fear and anger were observed as the dominant negative emotions that people had experienced (Lwin et al., 2020). According to a report by the World Health Organization (WHO, 2022), prevalence of anxiety and depression increased by 25% worldwide in the first year of the pandemic. Research (Han et al., 2020; Liu & Huang, 2020) reported that the broad spread of misinformation on COVID-19 was linked to emotions, anger in particular.

In addition to worsening the public's mental health, the proliferation of misinformation about COVID-19 also distorted people's risk judgment (Krause et al., 2020). When people believed that they were invulnerable to the disease, they were less likely to adopt preventative measures, including vaccinations. Other studies (Cheng & Luo, 2020; Liu & Huang, 2020; Yang & Yu, 2021) indicated that people tended to perceive others as more vulnerable to the negative impact of misinformation related to COVID-19 on social media.

Then, these questions arise. After encountering COVID-19 misinformation by virtue of exposure and sharing (refer to Chapters 3 and 4), what are the respondent's emotional responses to the infodemic about the virus? What is the role of exposure and sharing of misinformation in eliciting their negative emotions? In addition, how do they perceive their vulnerability to the impact of COVID-19 misinformation as compared to others? Will they display biased perception in believing the general public to be more impacted by the misinformation than themselves?

As the starting point of our comprehensive investigation of the public harm (i.e., adverse effects) of misinformation on respondents in Beijing, Hong Kong,

DOI: 10.4324/9781003355984-6

Singapore, and Taipei, we focus in this chapter on two major psychological consequences of misinformation exposure and sharing—negative emotions and biased risk perception of the harms of COVID-19 misinformation.

COVID-19 Misinformation, Negative Emotions and Risk Perception

As a crucial part of "sense making during crisis" (Tandoc & Lee, 2022, p. 783), emotions can shape individuals' perception of and response to health crises. According to cognitive appraisal theory, our evaluation of a situation will elicit emotional responses that are based on that appraisal (Lazarus, 1991; Lazarus & Smith, 1988). More importantly, negative emotions tend to occur when individuals face undesirable information that is incongruent with personal survival and well-being (Kim, 2015). Research has found that people have experienced various negative emotions during the pandemic, including fear, anger, anxiety, stress, and sadness (Lwin et al., 2020; Min et al., 2020; Wang & Zhang, 2022). In particular, fear and anger were the dominant emotions during the initial outbreaks partly due to the lack of sufficient knowledge about this virus and its potential harms (Lwin et al., 2020). Our big data analyses in Chapter 2 about the emergence of COVID-19 misinformation on Weibo as being closely related to the severity of the epidemic in China corroborate these studies. We also noted that rumormongers tended to choose the time when people were most panicked to spread misinformation, which further intensified public anxiety.

Emotions matter in understanding peoples' formation of attitudes and adoption of behaviors. Negative emotions aroused by exposure to misinformation can prompt attitudinal and behavioral changes. An online experiment (Featherstone & Zhang, 2020) revealed that exposure to vaccine misinformation generated anger among participants, which further decreased their pro-vaccination attitude. Another study found that emotional factors like guilt and anger motivated people to combat anti-vaccine misinformation (Sun et al., 2022b).

Furthermore, due to self-centered bias (Wei, 2020), people tend to presume different magnitudes of media effects on others relative to themselves during a public health crisis, leading to biased risk perceptions. The third-person hypothesis (Davison, 1983) states that people tend to believe that others are more likely to be influenced by media messages than themselves. The third-person perception concerning misinformation or disinformation related to COVID-19 and fake news on social media has been widely examined (Jang & Kim, 2018; Liu & Huang, 2020; Cheng & Luo, 2020). For example, Jang and Kim's research (2018) in the United States showed that Americans believed fake news would have greater effects on others than on themselves. Liu and Huang's study (2020) in China suggested that Chinese perceived themselves to be less susceptible to COVID-19 disinformation than were others. The greatest self-other discrepancy was found when Chinese people assessed the impacts of disinformation on social networking apps.

Grounded in the literature, this chapter examines multi-level factors that molded the respondents' emotions and shaped their biased risk perception during the first year of the pandemic. These factors included demographic variables (e.g., age, gender, and education), cognitive variables (e.g., elaboration), and societal variables (e.g., cities with different levels of access to digital information). Operationally, negative emotions elicited by COVID-19 misinformation were measured with four statements on a 5-point Likert scale: (1) I am worried about the possible consequences of COVID-19 misinformation; (2) I am annoyed with the possible consequences of COVID-19 misinformation; (3) I feel angry with the possible consequences of COVID-19 misinformation; and (4) I feel anxious about the possible consequences of COVID-19 misinformation. The items were averaged to create a composite index of negative emotions ($M = 3.69$, $SD = .80$, $\alpha = .85$).

Findings

Frequency analysis of the four emotion items about COVID-19 misinformation indicates that 4,094 respondents experienced moderate to strong negative emotions. Their strongest feeling was anger ($M = 3.76$, $SD = .98$), followed by annoyance ($M = 3.74$, $SD = .96$), worry ($M = 3.70$, $SD = .93$), and anxiety ($M = 3.56$, $SD = .99$) about the consequence of widely diffused misinformation in society.

Gender Differences in Negative Emotions

We first examined the consequences of exposure to misinformation on negative emotions. Through a series of t-test and ANOVA analyses, we compared the patterns of negative emotions by respondents' key demographic characteristics (i.e., gender, age, city of residence). Specifically, we conducted an independent sample t-test to explore if there were differences in overall and specific types of negative emotions by gender (male respondents = 1,978; female respondents = 2,116). No significant difference in overall negative emotions between male ($M = 3.71$, $SD = .83$) and female ($M = 3.67$, $SD = .78$) respondents ($t = 1.74$, $p > .05$) was found. Both men and women in the four cities held similar negative emotions elicited by the misinformation.

Among specific types of negative emotions associated with COVID-19 misinformation, male respondents ($M = 3.79$, $SD = .99$) reported a higher level of anger than their female counterparts ($M = 3.73$, $SD = .96$), $t = 2.08$, $p < .05$. No significant gender differences in worry ($t = 1.83$, $p > .05$), annoyance ($t = 1.42$, $p > .05$), and anxiety ($t = .52$, $p > .05$) existed.

Negative Emotions of Younger and Older Adults

To compare the respondents' negative emotions associated with COVID-19 misinformation by age, we split the age scale at the median to divide the younger (i.e., 18–39; n = 2,051) and older respondents (i.e., 40–85; n = 2,042) groups. The differences in overall negative emotions were not significant between younger (M = 3.71, SD = .78) and older respondents (M = 3.67, SD = .82), t = 1.63, p > .05.

In terms of specific negative emotions, compared to older respondents (M = 3.70, SD = .97), younger respondents (M = 3.78, SD = .96) exhibited a higher level of annoyance as a result of exposure to COVID-19 misinformation (t = 2.71, p < .01). There was no significant difference between younger and older respondents in feeling worried (t = 1.54, p > .05), angry (t = −.34, p > .05) and anxious (t = 1.55, p > .05).

Misinformation Exposure, Sharing, and Negative Emotions

To explore if respondents with different levels of misinformation exposure and sharing differed in their negative emotions, we split the misinformation exposure scale at the median to categorize the 4,094 respondents into low-exposure (n = 1,858) and high-exposure (n = 2,236) groups (for measures, refer to Chapter 4). Result of t-test analysis (see Table 6.1) indicated that respondents who had a high level of misinformation exposure (M = 3.81, SD = .72) experienced stronger overall negative emotions than those who had a low level of exposure (M =3.54, SD = .87) (t = −10.97, p < .001).

In addition, compared to respondents with low misinformation exposure, respondents with high misinformation exposure reported higher levels of worry (t = −6.04, p < .001), annoyance (t = −8.80, p < .001), anger (t = −10.7, p < .001) and anxiety (t= −10.7, p < .001). For respondents with high misinformation exposure, their most strongly experienced negative emotion was anger (M = 3.61, SD = .98); while those who had low misinformation exposure most strongly experienced worry (M = 3.90, SD = .91).

Following similar procedures, the respondents were divided into two groups by splitting the misinformation-sharing scale at the median, with 2,337 respondents being classified to the low-sharing group and 1,757 assigned to the high-sharing group (Chapter 5 has the scale and measures). As Table 6.2 shows, the low-sharing (M = 3.55, SD = .85) and high-sharing (M = 3.87, SD = .70) groups differed significantly in their overall negative emotions as a consequence of encountering COVID-19 misinformation on social media (t = −13.02, p < .001). That is, high-sharing respondents reported higher overall negative emotions compared to low-sharing respondents.

In terms of specific negative emotions, high-sharing respondents exhibited a higher level of worry (t = −7.51, p < .001), annoyance (t = −10.25, p < .001), anger (t = −9.89, p < .001), and anxiety (t = −15.34, p < .001) than

Table 6.1 Differences in negative emotions of COVID-19 misinformation between respondents of low and high misinformation exposure

	Low exposure (n = 1,858)	High exposure (n = 2,236)	
	M (SD)	M (SD)	t value
1 Worried about the possible consequences of COVID-19 misinformation	3.61 (.98)	3.78 (.87)	−6.04***
2 Annoyed with the possible consequences of COVID-19 misinformation	3.60 (1.01)	3.86 (.90)	−8.80***
3 Angry with the possible consequences of COVID-19 misinformation	3.58 (1.03)	3.90 (.91)	−10.70***
4 Anxious about the possible consequences of COVID-19 misinformation	3.38 (1.03)	3.70 (.93)	−10.70***
Combined index	3.54 (.87)	3.81 (.72)	−10.97***

Note: The items were rated from 1 to 5, where 1 = strongly disagree and 5 = strongly agree; ***$p < .001$.

Table 6.2 Differences in negative emotions of COVID-19 misinformation between respondents of low and high misinformation sharing

	Low sharing (n = 2,337)	High sharing (n = 1,757)	
	M (SD)	M (SD)	t value
1 Worried about the possible consequences of COVID-19 misinformation	3.61 (.97)	3.83 (.84)	−7.51***
2 Annoyed with the possible consequences of COVID-19 misinformation	3.61 (1.00)	3.92 (.88)	−10.25***
3 Angry with the possible consequences of COVID-19 misinformation	3.63 (1.01)	3.93 (.90)	−9.89***
4 Anxious about the possible consequences of COVID-19 misinformation	3.36 (1.02)	3.82 (.89)	−15.34***
Combined index	3.55 (.85)	3.87 (.70)	−13.02***

Note: The items were rated from 1 to 5, where 1 = strongly disagree and 5 = strongly agree; ***$p < .001$.

low-sharing respondents. For both low- and high-sharing respondents, their most strongly experienced negative emotion was anger ($M = 3.63$, $SD = 1.01$; $M = 3.93$, $SD = .90$ respectively).

Elaboration of Misinformation and Negative Emotions

To explore whether respondents with different levels of elaboration differed in their negative emotions, we created two groups by splitting the misinformation elaboration scale at the median. The low-elaboration group included 2,115 respondents and the high-elaboration group 1,979 respondents (the measures of elaboration can be found in Chapter 5). As presented in Table 6.3, in general, high-elaboration respondents ($M = 4.07$, $SD = .65$) experienced more negative emotions than low-elaboration respondents ($M = 3.33$, $SD = .77$) ($t = -32.92$, $p < .001$). That is, the more the respondents thought about the consequences of COVID-19 misinformation, the stronger their negative emotions were aroused.

Further, compared to high-elaboration respondents, low-elaboration respondents reported lower levels of worry ($t = -29.52$, $p < .001$), annoyance ($t = -27.01$, $p < .001$), anger ($t = -26.48$, $p < .001$), and anxiety ($t = -22.89$, $p < .001$). Respondents with low elaboration exhibited anger ($M = 3.40$, $SD = .96$) most strongly, whereas the most strongly negative emotions exhibited by high-elaboration respondents were annoyance ($M = 4.13$, $SD = .83$) and anger ($M = 4.14$, $SD = .84$).

City and Negative Emotions

A series of ANOVA was conducted to determine if there were any differences in negative emotions among respondents from the four culturally similar cities. Table 6.4 shows a significant difference in overall negative emotions

Table 6.3 Differences in negative emotions of COVID-19 misinformation between individuals of low level and highlevel of elaboration

	Low elaboration (n = 2,115)	High elaboration (n = 1,979)	
	M (SD)	M (SD)	t value
1 Worried about the possible consequences of COVID-19 misinformation	3.33 (.93)	4.11 (.73)	−29.52***
2 Annoyed with the possible consequences of COVID-19 misinformation	3.38 (.94)	4.13 (.83)	−27.01***
3 Angry with the possible consequences of COVID-19 misinformation	3.40 (.96)	4.14 (.84)	−26.48***
4 Anxious about the possible consequences of COVID-19 misinformation	3.23 (.94)	3.90 (.93)	−22.89***
Combined index	3.33 (.77)	4.07 (.65)	−32.92***

Note: The items were rated from 1 to 5, where 1 = strongly disagree and 5 = strongly agree; ***$p < .001$.

among respondents from the four cities, $F(3, 4090) = 105.84$, $p < .001$. Respondents from Beijing ($M = 3.96$, $SD = .70$) reported the highest level of overall negative emotions, followed by Singapore ($M = 3.80$, $SD = .79$), Taipei ($M = 3.62$, $SD = .80$), and Hong Kong ($M = 3.38$, $SD = .80$).

Beijing and Hong Kong respondents experienced anger the most strongly ($M = 4.10$, $SD = .87$; $M = 3.43$, $SD = .93$ respectively). While Taipei respondents experienced annoyance ($M = 3.69$, $SD = .93$) as well as anger ($M = 3.69$, $SD = .97$) the most strongly. For Singapore respondents, the strongest negative emotion elicited by misinformation was annoyance ($M = 3.93$, $SD = .91$). This cross-societal result makes sense because Beijing respondents had a higher level of exposure to misinformation, which elicited the strongest negative emotions.

Predictors of Negative Emotions

Further, to identify the significant predictors of negative emotions, we performed a hierarchical regression to examine the effects of control variables

Table 6.4 Differences in negative emotions among respondents in Beijing, Hong Kong, Taipei, and Singapore

	Beijing (n = 1,033)	Hong Kong (n = 1,017)	Taipei (n = 1,019)	Singapore (n = 1,025)	Total	F value
1 Worried about the possible consequences of COVID-19 misinformation	3.90 (.86)	3.42 (.92)	3.67 (.94)	3.82 (.92)	3.70 (.93)	56.02***
2 Annoyed with the possible consequences of COVID-19 misinformation	3.96 (.90)	3.39 (1.00)	3.69 (.93)	3.93 (.91)	3.74 (.96)	81.44***
3 Angry with the possible consequences of COVID-19 misinformation	4.10 (.87)	3.43 (.93)	3.69 (.97)	3.80 (.98)	3.76 (.98)	85.92***
4 Anxious about the possible consequences of COVID-19 misinformation	3.86 (.94)	3.27 (.97)	3.42 (1.00)	3.66 (.96)	3.56 (.99)	75.48***
Combined index	3.96 (.70)	3.38 (.80)	3.62 (.80)	3.80 (.79)	3.69 (.80)	105.84***

Note: The items were rated from 1 to 5, where 1 = strongly disagree and 5 = strongly agree; ***$p < .001$

(e.g., demographics), media use, misinformation-related variables (e.g., exposure, sharing, and elaboration). Results shown in Table 6.5 revealed the predictive power of demographics. City of residence was a positive predictor of negative emotions (β = .08, p < .001). Respondents from Beijing also reported significantly higher levels of negative emotions.

When the influences of the control variables were taken into account, use of newspapers (β = .08, p < .001), TV (β = .04, p < .05), and use of social media for news (β = .08, p < .001) were significant and positive predictors of negative emotions, suggesting the more media use, the stronger negative emotions they elicited. In addition, misinformation exposure (β = .06, p < .001) and misinformation sharing (β = .07, p < .001) were significantly related to negative emotions as well. Moreover, among all the independent variables, elaboration of misinformation turned out to be the strongest predictor of negative emotions (β = .51, p < .001). It alone accounted for 21.7% of the variance in the dependent variable.

Taken together, these results indicate that exposure to and sharing of misinformation resulted in stronger negative emotions. Thinking about the consequence of misinformation pushed anger, anxiety, annoyance, and worry to even higher levels.

Table 6.5 Hierarchical regression analysis predicting negative emotions

Predictors	Negative emotions
Block 1: Demographics	
Age	.02
Gender (Male = 1)	–.00
Education	–.02
City (Beijing = 1)	.08***
Adjusted R^2	4.1%
Block 2: Media use	
Newspapers	.08***
TV news	.04*
Online news	.02
Social media news	.08***
Incremental adjusted R^2	9.6%
Block 3: Misinformation exposure	
Misinformation exposure	.06***
Incremental adjusted R^2	2.5%
Block 4: Misinformation sharing	
Misinformation sharing	.07***
Incremental adjusted R^2	0.7%
Block 5: Elaboration	
Elaboration	.51***
Incremental adjusted R^2	21.7%
Total adjusted R^2	38.8%

Note: N = 4,093; Beijing was coded as 1 and other cities were coded as 0; ***p < .001; The age entry has one missing value.

Gender and Perceived Influence of Misinformation

Next, we explored the relationships between respondents' demographics, misinformation-related variables, negative emotions, and perceived influence of misinformation. The measurement of perceived influence of COVID-19 misinformation on others relied on three items about respondents' estimate of the influence of misinformation on the general public's (1) understanding of the current COVID-19 situation; (2) understanding of the major developments of the pandemic; and (3) knowledge about the COVID-19 virus. The response categories ranged from "1" (no influence at all) to "5" (a great deal of influence). The three items were averaged to form an index of perceived influence on others ($M = 3.53$, $SD = .81$, $\alpha = .89$). Using the same statements, the perceived influence on self was measured by replacing the public with "I." Another composite measure was formed by averaging the items. ($M = 3.02$, $SD = .99$, $\alpha = .90$). The measure of third-person perception was derived from substituting the means of on self from that on others ($M = .51$, $SD = .93$).

We found that biased perception of influence of misinformation related to COVID-19 existed. Based on the mean score of perceived influence on others ($M = 3.53$, $SD = .81$) and on self ($M = 3.02$, $SD = .99$), respondents tended to believe others to be more influenced by the misinformation than themselves.

To explore gender difference in perceived influence of COVID-19 misinformation on self and others, we ran a series of t-test analyses. Results showed that both male and female respondents perceived misinformation to have greater influence on others than on themselves. However, the third-person effect differentials (third-person perception, TPP) were not significant between male and female respondents in their perceived effects of misinformation on COVID-19 current situation understanding ($t = 1.70$, $p > .05$), major developments understanding ($t = .96$, $p > .05$), knowledge ($t = 1.96$, $p > .05$), and the combined index ($t = 1.80$, $p > .05$).

Age and Perceived Influence of Misinformation

Respondents were classified into younger (i.e., 18–39; $n = 2,051$) and older groups (i.e., 40–85, $n = 2,042$) by splitting the age scale at the median. Results of t-test analyses in Table 6.6 showed that both younger and older respondents tended to perceive that others were more influenced by misinformation than they themselves in the pooled sample. The same pattern also applied to the perceived effects of misinformation on COVID-19 current situation understanding, major developments understanding, and knowledge.

The third-person effect differentials were also significant between younger and older respondents in their perceived effects of misinformation on COVID-19 current situation understanding ($t = 3.60$, $p < .001$), major developments understanding ($t = 2.58$, $p < .01$), knowledge ($t = 2.29$, $p < .01$), and the combined index ($t = 3.28$, $p < .001$). These results indicate that older respondents tend to have significantly larger third-person perceptions than their younger counterparts.

Table 6.6 Differences in perceived effects of COVID-19 misinformation on self and others between younger and older adults

	Younger adults (n = 2,051)			Older adults (n = 2,042)			
	Self	Others	TPP	Self	Others	TPP	t value
1 Understanding of the current situation of COVID-19 pandemic	3.12 (.99)	3.53 (.85)	.41 (1.02)	2.87 (1.06)	3.40 (.87)	.52 (1.05)	3.60***
2 Understanding of the COVID-19 pandemic's major developments	3.18 (1.05)	3.64 (.91)	.46 (1.08)	2.90 (1.11)	3.45 (.90)	.54 (1.08)	2.58**
3 Knowledge about COVID-19 virus	3.16 (1.09)	3.67 (.94)	.51 (1.11)	2.90 (1.13)	3.48 (.92)	.59 (1.11)	2.29*
Combined index	3.15 (.93)	3.61 (.79)	.46 (.91)	2.89 (1.02)	3.44 (.81)	.55 (.95)	3.28***

Note: The items were rated from 1 to 5, where 1 = not influential at all and 5 = extremely influential; $*p < .05$, $**p < .01$, $***p < .001$.

Misinformation Exposure, Sharing, and Perceived Influence of Misinformation

To examine how people with different levels of exposure to misinformation differed in their perceived influence on self and others, more t-test analyses were conducted. Misinformation exposure scale was split at the median to divide the low-exposure ($n = 1,858$) and high-exposure ($n = 2,236$) groups. Results in Table 6.7 of t-tests show that both high-exposure and low-exposure respondents tended to believe misinformation to have greater influence on others than on themselves. Results also show that respondents with low-exposure ($M = .59$, $SD = .97$) reported higher overall third-person perception scores than high-exposure ($M = .44$, $SD = .89$) respondents ($t = 5.10$, $p < .001$). Moreover, compared to high-exposure respondents, low-exposure respondents also perceived higher third-person perception on their own COVID-19 current situation understanding ($t = 4.85$, $p < .001$), major developments understanding ($t = 4.00$, $p < .001$), and knowledge ($t = 4.26$, $p < .001$).

Regarding COVID-19 sharing of misinformation and perceived influence, we split the misinformation-sharing scale at the median to classify respondents into low-sharing ($n = 2,337$) and high-sharing ($n = 1,757$) groups. As illustrated in Table 6.8, both low-sharing and high-sharing respondents perceived misinformation to have greater influence on others than on themselves. Compared to high-sharing respondents ($M = .24$, $SD = .74$), low-sharing ($M = .70$, $SD = 1.00$) respondents exhibited higher overall third-person perception ($t = 12.07$, $p < .001$). Low-sharing respondents also demonstrated

Table 6.7 Differences in perceived effects of COVID-19 misinformation on self and others between individuals of low and high misinformation exposure

	Low exposure (n = 1,858)			High exposure (n = 2,236)			
	Self	Others	TPP	Self	Others	TPP	t value
1 Understanding of the current situation of COVID-19 pandemic	2.78 (1.05)	3.33 (.89)	.56 (1.07)	3.17 (.98)	3.57 (.84)	.40 (1.00)	4.85***
2 Understanding of the COVID-19 pandemic's major developments	2.81 (1.08)	3.38 (.91)	.57 (1.07)	3.24 (1.05)	3.68 (.89)	.44 (1.08)	4.00***
3 Knowledge about COVID-19 virus	2.77 (1.10)	3.40 (.97)	.63 (1.11)	3.24 (1.08)	3.72 (.88)	.59 (.99)	4.26***
Combined index	2.79 (1.01)	3.37 (.85)	.59 (.97)	3.22 (.92)	3.66 (.74)	.44 (.89)	5.10***

Note: The items were rated from 1 to 5, where 1 = not influential at all and 5 = extremely influential; *p < .05, **p < .01, ***p < .001.

Table 6.8 Differences in perceived effects of COVID-19 misinformation on self and others between individuals of low and high misinformation sharing

	Low sharing (n = 2,337)			High sharing (n = 1,757)			
	Self	Others	TPP	Self	Others	TPP	t value
1 Understanding of the current situation of COVID-19 pandemic	2.68 (1.00)	3.37 (.89)	.69 (1.08)	3.41 (.92)	3.58 (.82)	.17 (.90)	−16.78***
2 Understanding of the COVID-19 pandemic's major developments	2.71 (1.03)	3.40 (.92)	.68 (1.11)	3.48 (1.00)	3.73 (.86)	.25 (.99)	13.10***
3 Knowledge about COVID-19 virus	2.71 (1.07)	3.45 (.95)	.74 (1.17)	3.45 (1.02)	3.75 (.88)	.29 (1.01)	12.96***
Combined index	2.70 (.96)	3.41 (.85)	.70 (1.00)	3.45 (.85)	3.69 (.71)	.24 (.74)	12.07***

Note: The items were rated from 1 to 5, where 1 = not influential at all and 5 = extremely influential; ***p < .001.

higher third-person perception of misinformation on COVID-19 current situation understanding ($t = 16.78$, $p < .001$), major developments understanding ($t = 13.10$, $p < .001$), and knowledge ($t = 12.96$, $p < .001$).

Elaboration and Perceived Influence of Misinformation

To explore the relationship between elaboration of COVID-19 misinformation and perceived influence, the misinformation elaboration scale was split at the median to distinguish respondents into low-elaboration (*n* = 2,115) and high-elaboration (*n* = 1,979) groups. Result of a t-test analysis shown in Table 6.9 indicates that both groups believed misinformation to have greater influence on others than on themselves. In addition, high-elaboration respondents (*M* = .58, *SD* = .99) reported higher overall third-person perception than low-elaboration respondents (*M* = .43, *SD* = .86). Furthermore, compared to low-elaboration respondents, high-elaboration respondents also revealed higher third-person perception on COVID-19 current situation understanding (*t* = 5.89, *p* < .001), major developments understanding (*t* = 3.08, *p* < .01), and knowledge (*t* = 4.64, *p* < .001) than low-elaboration respondents.

Such patterns are consistent with the findings concerning the relationships between exposure to and sharing of misinformation and perceived influence. In general, the greater exposure to, sharing of, and elaboration of misinformation, the greater the perceived effects on others and on self.

Negative Emotions and Perceived Influence of Misinformation

To explore if negative emotions elicited by COVID-19 misinformation affect perceived influence, we split negative emotions scale at the median to generate two groups: respondents into low-negative emotions (*n* = 1,678) and high-negative emotions (*n* = 2,416) groups. As Table 6.10 shows, respondents in both groups perceived that misinformation influenced others more

Table 6.9 Differences in perceived effects of COVID-19 misinformation on self and others between individuals of low and high level of elaboration

	Low elaboration (n = 2,115)			High elaboration (n = 1,979)			
	Self	Others	TPP	Self	Others	TPP	t value
1 Understanding of the current situation of COVID-19 pandemic	2.80 (.93)	3.18 (.81)	.38 (.99)	3.20 (1.09)	3.77 (.82)	.57 (1.08)	5.89***
2 Understanding of the COVID-19 pandemic's major developments	2.83 (.96)	3.28 (.85)	.45 (1.01)	3.27 (1.16)	3.83 (.89)	.55 (1.15)	3.08**
3 Knowledge about COVID-19 virus	2.83 (1.00)	3.29 (.88)	.47 (1.06)	3.25 (1.18)	3.88 (.90)	.63 (1.19)	4.64***
Combined index	2.82 (.86)	3.25 (.74)	.43 (.86)	3.24 (1.06)	3.82 (.77)	.58 (.99)	5.27***

Note: The items were rated from 1 to 5, where 1 = not influential at all and 5 = extremely influential; **p* < .01, ****p* < .001.

Table 6.10 Differences in perceived effects of COVID-19 misinformation on self and others between individuals of low and high negative emotion

	Low negative emotion (n = 1,678)			High negative emotion (n = 2,416)			
	Self	*Others*	*TPP*	*Self*	*Others*	*TPP*	*t value*
1 Understanding of the current situation of COVID-19 pandemic	2.66 (.92)	3.12 (.83)	.46 (1.00)	3.22 (1.04)	3.70 (.82)	.47 (1.06)	.25
2 Understanding of the COVID-19 pandemic's major developments	2.69 (.94)	3.20 (.85)	.51 (1.03)	3.29 (1.12)	3.78 (.88)	.49 (1.11)	.60
3 Knowledge about COVID-19 virus	2.68 (.98)	3.22 (.87)	.54 (1.08)	3.27 (1.13)	3.82 (.90)	.55 (1.16)	.35
Combined index	2.68 (.85)	3.18 (.75)	.51 (.90)	3.26 (1.00)	3.77 (.76)	.51 (.95)	.00

Note: The items were rated from 1 to 5, where 1 = not influential at all and 5 = extremely influential.

than themselves. However, the overall third-person perception between the two groups was not significant ($t = 0.00$, $p > .05$). Further, there was no difference between the third-person perception of the two groups with respect to COVID-19 current situation understanding ($t= .25$, $p > .05$), major developments understanding ($t = .60$, $p > .05$), and knowledge ($t = .35$, $p > .05$). All of the differences were not significant, indicating negative emotions due to exposure to misinformation did not lead to greater third-person perception.

City and Perceived Influence of Misinformation

We conducted a series of ANOVA to find out if respondents in Beijing, Hong Kong, Taipei, and Singapore differed in their presumed influence of COVID-19 misinformation on self and others. As indicated in Table 6.11, respondents from the four cities tended to perceive that others were more influenced by misinformation than themselves. Further, the overall third-person perception was significant, $F(3, 4090) = 42.29$, $p < .001$. The highest third-person perception was reported by Taipei respondents ($M = .74$, $SD = 1.01$), followed by respondents from Hong Kong ($M = .55$, $SD = .91$), Singapore ($M = .43$, $SD = .95$), and Beijing ($M = .30$, $SD = .76$).

Regarding the perceived influence on others, respondents from the four cities also exhibited a significant difference in their overall perceived influence on others, $F(3, 4090) = 45.41$, $p < .001$. Beijing respondents ($M = 3.69$, $SD = .77$) again reported the highest level of overall perceived effects on others, followed by Taipei ($M = 3.62$, $SD = .77$), Hong Kong ($M = 3.49$, $SD = .77$), and Singapore ($M = 3.31$, $SD = .86$).

Table 6.11 Differences in perceived effects of COVID-19 misinformation on self, perceived effects on others among Beijing, Hong Kong, Taipei, and Singapore

	Beijing (n = 1,033)			Hong Kong (n = 1,017)			Taipei (n = 1,019)			Singapore (n = 1,025)			F value
	Self	Others	TPP	Self	Others	TPP	Self	Others	TPP	Self	Others	TPP	
1 Understanding of the current situation of COVID-19 pandemic	3.33 (1.01)	3.62 (.86)	.29 (.95)	2.93 (.89)	3.42 (.84)	.49 (1.00)	2.87 (1.02)	3.55 (.83)	.68 (1.10)	2.84 (1.11)	3.26 (.90)	.43 (1.06)	25.86 ***
2 Understanding of the COVID-19 pandemic's major developments	3.43 (1.08)	3.73 (.92)	.30 (1.02)	2.97 (.98)	3.51 (.88)	.54 (1.08)	2.88 (1.04)	3.62 (.83)	.74 (1.09)	2.89 (1.15)	3.30 (.94)	.41 (1.08)	32.13 ***
3 Knowledge about COVID-19 virus	3.39 (1.13)	3.72 (.95)	.32 (1.04)	2.94 (.99)	3.55 (.92)	.61 (1.10)	2.88 (1.08)	3.68 (.87)	.80 (1.19)	2.90 (1.16)	3.35 (.96)	.46 (1.12)	34.87 ***
Combined index	3.38 (.95)	3.69 (.77)	.30 (.76)	2.95 (.85)	3.49 (.77)	.55 (.91)	2.88 (.97)	3.62 (.77)	.74 (1.01)	2.87 (1.07)	3.31 (.86)	.43 (.95)	42.29 ***

Note: The items were rated from 1 to 5, where 1 = not influential at all and 5 = extremely influential; ***p < .001.

Predicting Perceived Influence of Misinformation

Finally, with the purpose of identifying the significant predictors of perceived effects on self, perceived effects on others, and third-person perception, three hierarchical regression analyses were performed. The predictor variables were control variables (e.g., demographics), media use, misinformation-related variables (e.g., exposure sharing and elaboration), and negative emotions.

Table 6.12 (see the first column) presents the regression results. In predicting presumed influence on self, age (β = −.10, p < .001) was a negative predictor. That is, respondents who were younger would acknowledge the influence of misinformation on themselves. In contrast, city of residence (β = .08, p < .001) was a positive predictor of the dependent variable. In addition, the media use block had three significant predictors, including reading newspapers (β = .05, p < .001), viewing TV news (β = .04, p < .01), and reading news online (β = −.06, p < .001). In other words, respondents who lived in Beijing and had a more frequent use of newspapers and TV news tended to perceive a higher influence of COVID-19 misinformation on self. In contrast,

Table 6.12 Hierarchical regression analyses predicting perceived effects of COVID-19 misinformation on self and others

Predictors	Perceived effects on self	Perceived effects on others	TPP
Block 1: Demographics			
Age	−.10***	−.05***	.05**
Gender (Male = 1)	−.02	−.01	.02
Education	−.01	.04**	.05**
City (Beijing=1)	.08***	−.00	−.08***
Adjusted R²	6.1%	2.9%	2.3%
Block 2: Media use			
Newspapers	.05***	−.01	−.07***
TV news	.04**	.08***	.03
Online news	−.06***	.02	.08***
Social media news	.02	.01	−.02
Incremental adjusted R²	5.5%	4.6%	2.5%
Block 3: Misinformation exposure			
Misinformation exposure	.13***	.12***	−.03
Incremental adjusted R²	5.7%	4.0%	0.6%
Block 4: Misinformation sharing			
Misinformation sharing	.29***	.05***	−.26***
Incremental adjusted R²	7.5%	0.5%	5.0%
Block 5: Elaboration			
Elaboration	.04*	.24***	.17***
Incremental adjusted R²	1.8%	10.3%	1.9%
Block 6: Negative emotions			
Negative emotions	.21***	.21***	−.04*
Incremental adjusted R²	2.7%	2.7%	0.0%
Total adjusted R²	29.3%	25.0%	12.3%

Note: N = 4,093; Beijing was coded as 1 and other cities were coded as 0; ***p < .001; The age entry has one missing value.

older respondents with a higher level of online news use tended to perceive a lower influence of COVID-19 misinformation on self.

It is worth noting that exposure to misinformation (β = .13, p < .001), sharing of misinformation (β = .29, p < .001), elaboration of misinformation (β = .04, p < .05) as well as negative emotions (β = .21, p < .001) positively predicted perceived influence on self. They added predictive power over the dependent variable. In fact, sharing of misinformation was the strongest predictor, followed by negative emotions and misinformation exposure. These results indicate that higher level of exposure to and sharing of misinformation led to greater perceived influence of COVID-19 misinformation on self. The higher the negative emotions, the greater the perceived influence as well.

Following the same steps, we ran a separate regression with perceived influence of misinformation on others as the second dependent variable. As results in Table 6.12 show (the second column), age was a negative predictor of the perceived influence on others (β = −.05, p < .001). That is, younger respondents tended to perceive greater influence on other people. Although not a significant predictor of perceived influence on self, education positively predicted perceived influence on others (β = .04, p < .001). However, city of residence, (β = −.00, p > .05) was not a significant predictor of presumed influence on others. Respondents in Beijing did not perceive more influence on others.

Regarding the effects of media use, viewing TV news (β = .08, p < .001) was a positive predictor of the perceived influence on others. Respondents who viewed TV news more frequently perceived a greater influence on others.

Additionally, misinformation exposure (β = .12, p < .001), misinformation sharing (β = .05, p < .001), elaboration (β = .24, p < .001), and negative emotions (β = .21, p < .001) also positively predicted the perceived influence on others. That is, respondents with a higher level of exposure to, sharing of, and elaboration of misinformation tended to perceive a greater influence on others, which is consistent with the findings concerning the perceived influence on self. Negative emotions were also significantly related to perceived influence on others.

Finally, to explore the significant predictors of third-person perception, we ran a third hierarchical regression. As shown in Table 6.12 (see the third column), age (β = .05, p < .01) and education (β = .05, p < .01) positively predicted third-person perception, whereas city of residence (β = −.08, p < .001) was a negative predictor. In addition, the media use block had two significant predictors, including reading newspapers (β = −.07, p < .001) and reading news online (β = .08, p < .001). In other words, older respondents with higher education tended to have a greater third-person perception regarding the presumed influence of misinformation. In contrast, respondents who lived in Beijing who reported a more frequent use of newspapers tended to show a smaller third-person perception.

Moreover, sharing of misinformation (β = −.26, p < .001), elaboration of misinformation (β = .17, p < .001), as well as negative emotions (β = −.04,

$p < .05$) significantly predicted third-person perception. In fact, sharing of misinformation was the strongest predictor, followed by elaboration. These results indicate that a higher level of misinformation sharing and negative emotions led to smaller third-person perception of presumed influence of COVID-19 misinformation. The higher the elaboration, the greater the biased perception.

Summary of Key Findings

This chapter focused on exploring the patterns and mechanisms underlying the links between misinformation and negative emotions as well as risk perception among the 4,094 respondents we surveyed in the four cities. Results indicated that the negative emotions and perception of the influence of misinformation were accounted for by demographic characteristics, media use patterns, and encountering misinformation related to COVID-19. In general, the greater levels of exposure to, sharing of, and elaboration of misinformation, the stronger negative emotions and biased perceptions. To be specific:

• No gender or age difference exited in the overall negative emotions elicited by COVID-19 misinformation. Men and women, young and old, all held negative emotions elicited by the misinformation. Their strongest feeling was anger whereas the weakest was anxiety.
• Levels of exposure to, sharing of, and elaboration of misinformation made a difference in respondents' feelings about the possible harmful impact of misinformation. Respondents who had high-misinformation exposure reported stronger overall negative emotions than did respondents with low-misinformation exposure. Consistently, high-sharing respondents reported stronger overall negative emotion than low-sharing respondents. In addition, the same pattern was found with levels of elaboration about misinformation, which turned out to be the strongest predictor of negative emotions. That is, thinking about the possible consequences of misinformation made respondents anxious, angry, annoyed, and worried.
• Among the respondents in the four cities, Beijing respondents reported the highest level of overall negative emotions, followed by those from Singapore, Taipei, and Hong Kong. This pattern may result from different levels of exposure to the misinformation as discussed in Chapter 4.
• With regard to perceptions about influence of misinformation, younger respondents presumed a greater influence on themselves and on others than did older respondents.
• Respondents with high exposure to and high sharing of COVID-19 misinformation tended to perceive great overall influence on self and others than those with low exposure and low sharing. Additionally, high-elaboration respondents rated higher overall perceived influence on self and others than that of low-elaboration respondents. These results underscore that a higher level of encountering and thinking about the possible harms of COVID-19 misinformation may lead to greater perception of the influence.

- Respondents from Beijing, Hong Kong, Taipei, and Singapore exhibited significant differences in perceiving the influence of COVID-19 misinformation on self and others. Beijing respondents self-reported the highest level of overall perceived effects on self and perceived effects on others, and those in Singapore had the lowest.

Qualitative Findings

Anger, Annoyance, and Coping

Participants in the focus groups revealed why some were angrier or more annoyed than others about COVID-related misinformation. Beijing and Hong Kong residents experienced anger the most, while Taipei and Singaporean residents felt annoyance the most. Anger exploded on social media in China during the initial stage of the outbreaks, then gradually diminished (Li et al., 2020). According to the accounts of the participants from Beijing, anger was not an individual matter but rather was associated with or even produced by a broader social context, especially the "social hostility" that diffused widely throughout online channels. As a young male informant from Beijing, Mr. Huang explained,

> the social hostility phenomenon does not just happen on the Internet. Actually, in our society, people are becoming more hostile to each other. Sometimes, just within a few sentences, people start to 'battle' you... [Sometimes when there is fake news], and if you tell the netizen that this is fake, they probably won't believe you, or worse, they will argue with you, and eventually it becomes a fight.

In comparison, participants from Hong Kong seemed to be angry at the contents of the rumors and misleading information. Some rumors were actually the same stuff recycled from the SARS epidemic in 2003. A young male participant Elijah who was born around the time of SARS still remembered such rumors and felt it was ridiculous that they could still be prevalent almost two decades later. He said,

> What impressed me the most was, at the beginning [of the COVID-19 pandemic], I don't know why, but someone mentioned Banlangen (Indigowoad root, a type of Chinese herbal medicine), saying that it can be used to treat COVID. How stupid! It's already 2020! In 2003, medical specialists and the news media had told you that there was no scientific basis [to say Banlangen can treat SARS]. Later, I also received messages, for no reasons, saying that it [Banlangen] could be effective... I think, wow, it seems like people are not yet enlightened....

It seemed worthless or pointless to participants from Taipei and Singapore to be too emotionally attached to the misinformation. They felt upset but would not allow the negative emotions to "stick." Camila, a female heavy user of social media from Singapore, developed her own coping strategy for the negativity growing from misinformation. She explained,

> I've also heard of fake news like that... But this kind of things, I think... it's more like a debate, kind of like a topic to talk amongst your family and your friends... when I hear such news, obviously I'll be a bit upset, like why would people want to do this kind of thing for the world? But then I wouldn't let it linger for too long because what can I do?... the most I can do is to stay upset but I cannot change anything. And so I'll just try not to think about it and just try to move on and think about how we can fight the virus instead. So, at first, when I heard about it, I'll be like angry. I'm like, why? Why would people do that? But then I wouldn't let it bother me too much.

Ms. Chuang, a 58-year-old female housekeeper from Taiwan, moved one step forward. Instead of letting the negative emotions aroused by the misinformation get in her way, she said she would read or watch something more cheerful.

To cope with the negative emotions elicited from viewing or reading fake news or misinformation about COVID-19, a good number of the participants revealed that they chose to participate less in online or offline discussions of the pandemic, engaging in a sort of "information avoidance." Levi, a male Chinese Singaporean, attributed avoiding discussing or arguing with others about fake news to Chinese culture. As he remarked,

> We know really what is false and what is true. And I also point out that we are actually very traditional. I mean, as for me, I'm actually a very traditional Chinese family. There's really no way that you can talk to your elders or talk to your seniors in this manner, right? I mean to a certain extent even you know that there's fake news, you can't really tell them in the face that you know, 'Hey, uncle, hey, aunty, this is bad'. Yeah, due to our upbring as Chinese. I mean, yeah, I know about your culture back there, but over here, it's you can't talk back to your seniors per se.

What is conveyed here is more than just filial piety or respect for elders. Levi's example also demonstrates that when encountering undesirable content, people will think about others, especially those who are more vulnerable, less knowledgeable, and more susceptible to the content (Sun et al., 2008). A 36-year-old female participant Ms. Cheng from Taipei told the story of her parents' quarrel over the "authenticity" of news about the lockdowns in Shanghai in Spring 2022. In her account,

> The most ridiculous thing I have ever heard is from my parents – they like to quarrel very much – about the news from China. I know that

during the lockdowns in Shanghai, many people had nothing to eat. Some communities might have many supplies, but since no one can deliver, they all got rotten. But the news my parents received was that Shanghai people had too much food to eat, and that the CCP did a very good job; that is, everyone had food to eat during the lockdowns. This is the most amazing [rumor] I've ever heard. It seems to turn black into white... I don't know where they got it from.

It's the Information Age

When the discussion among the focus groups participants involved their own emotional response to COVID-19 misinformation, a number claimed that they were less affected by the spread of the misinformation. A 54-year-old male education institution manager in Beijing Mr. He said something like this to describe his non-emotional approach to misinformation,

It's the information age now; information is transparent and updated quickly. If it's fake, it's fake. If he or she wants to post it, he/she'll post it. By no means will I pass it on. That's the end of story. It [misinformation] didn't have any effect on me. I will just laugh it off and read it as if it's a joke.

A recent study (Han et al., 2020) suggests that to deal with their anger, people may believe in and spread COVID-related misinformation even more. As such, angry citizens may experience more exposure, more sharing, and more information elaboration, which further reinforces their anger. The next chapter further explores the complicated relationships between encounters with misinformation and attitudes.

Conclusion and Insights

Our findings in this chapter lead to some insights concerning respondents' emotional responses to and perceptions of COVID-19 misinformation in society:

First, misleading and factually incorrect information about the coronavirus has indeed elicited negative emotions among the general public. It makes people angry, worried, anxious, and annoyed. The more they encounter such misinformation on social media, the stronger their negative emotions, which adds to the woes on the public's mental well-being caused by the disease. Thus, the emotional cost of misinformation should be taken into account in fully understanding its harms in society. To protect citizens' psychological well-being during a pandemic, government and public health officials should make a major effort to combat misinformation by providing factual and evidence-based information that will help the public to fact-check and debunk false or inaccurate information.

Second, respondents in our study tended to perceive a greater influence of misinformation on others than on themselves. The greater the encounter by virtue of exposure and sharing, the smaller the third-person perception. More importantly, elaboration was a key cognitive mechanism in shaping respondents' misinformation processing; the more respondents thought about the possible consequences of COVID-19 misinformation, the greater influence they presumed on themselves and on others, the greater the third-person perception. Taking these patterns together with those of emotional response, the perceived harms of misinformation on other citizens were attenuated by exposure to and sharing of the misinformation, but they were enhanced by thinking deeply about the consequences of the misinformation.

Finally, another major insight gained from this chapter is that the impacts of COVID-19 misinformation appeared to be differential across the four societies in our study. We found that Beijing respondents reported the highest level of overall negative emotions and perceived effects on themselves and on others largely due to their greater exposure to COVID-19 misinformation. Thus, structural differences in controlling access and exposure to misinformation play a critical role in protecting citizens' mental well-being and reducing their biased perception.

References

Cheng, Y., & Luo, Y. (2020). The presumed influence of digital misinformation: Examining US public's support for governmental restrictions versus corrective action in the COVID-19 pandemic. *Online Information Review, 45*(4), 834–852. https://doi.org/10.1108/oir-08-2020-0386

Davison, W. P. (1983). The third-person effect in communication. *Public Opinion Quarterly, 47*(1), 1–15.

Featherstone, J. D., & Zhang, J. (2020). Feeling angry: The effects of vaccine misinformation and refutational messages on negative emotions and vaccination attitude. *Journal of Health Communication, 25*(9), 692–702. https://doi.org/10.1080/10810730.2020.1838671

Han, J., Cha, M., & Lee, W. (2020). Anger contributes to the spread of COVID-19 misinformation. *Harvard Kennedy School Misinformation Review, 1*(3), 1–14. https://doi.org/10.37016/mr-2020-39

Jang, S. M., & Kim, J. K. (2018). Third person effects of fake news: Fake news regulation and media literacy interventions. *Computers in Human Behavior, 80,* 295–302. https://doi.org/10.1016/j.chb.2017.11.034

Kim, H. (2015). Perception and emotion: The indirect effect of reported election poll results on political participation intention and support for restrictions. *Mass Communication and Society, 18*(3), 303–324. https://doi.org/10.1080/15205436.2014.945650

Krause, N. M., Freiling, I., Beets, B., & Brossard, D. (2020). Fact-checking as risk communication: The multi-layered risk of misinformation in times of COVID-19. *Journal of Risk Research*, 1–8. https://doi.org/10.1080/13669877.2020.1756385

Lazarus, R. (1991). *Emotion and adaptation.* New York, NY: Oxford University Press.

Lazarus, R., & Smith, C. (1988). Knowledge and appraisal in the cognition-emotion relationship. *Cognition & Emotion, 2,* 281–300. https://doi.org/10.1080/02699938808412701

Li, X., Zhou, M., Wu, J., et al. (2020). Analyzing COVID-19 on online social media: Trends, sentiments and emotions. *ArXiv:2005.14464* [Cs]. http://arxiv.org/abs/2005.14464.

Liu, P. L., & Huang, L. V. (2020). Digital disinformation about COVID-19 and the third-person effect: Examining the channel differences and negative emotional outcomes. *Cyberpsychology, Behavior, and Social Networking, 23*(11), 789–793. https://doi.org/10.1089/cyber.2020.0363

Lwin, M. O., Lu, J., Sheldenkar, A., Schulz, P. J., Shin, W., Gupta, R., et al. (2020). Global sentiments surrounding the COVID-19 pandemic on Twitter: Analysis of Twitter trends. *JMIR Public Health Surveillance, 6*(2), Article e19447. https://doi.org/10.2196/19447

Min, C., Shen, F., Yu, W., & Chu, Y. (2020). The relationship between government trust and preventive behaviors during the COVID-19 pandemic in China: Exploring the roles of knowledge and negative emotion. *Preventive Medicine, 141,* Article 106288. https://doi.org/10.1016/j.ypmed.2020.106288

Pfefferbaum, B., & North, C. S. (2020). Mental health and the Covid-19 pandemic. *The New England Journal of Medicine, 383*(6), 510–512. https://doi.org/10.1056/NEJMp2008017

Ridder, J. (2021). What's so bad about misinformation? *Inquiry,* 1–23. https://doi.org/10.1080/0020174X.2021.2002187

Sun, Y., Oktavianus, J., Wang, S., & Lu, F. (2022b). The role of influence of presumed influence and anticipated guilt in evoking social correction of COVID-19 misinformation. *Health Communication, 37*(11), 1368–1377. https://doi.org/10.1080/10410236.2021.1888452

Sun, Y., Pan, Z., & Shen, L. (2008). Understanding the third-person perception: Evidence from a meta-analysis. *Journal of Communication, 58*(2), 280–300. https://doi.org/10.1111/j.1460-2466.2008.00385.x

Tandoc, Jr., E., & Lee, J. (2022). When viruses and misinformation spread: How young Singaporeans navigated uncertainty in the early stages of the COVID-19 outbreak. *New Media & Society, 24*(3), 778–796. https://doi.org/10.1177/1461444820968212

Wang, R., & Zhang, H. (2022). Who spread COVID-19 (mis) information online? Differential informedness, psychological mechanisms, and intervention strategies. *Computers in Human Behavior,* 107486. https://doi.org/10.1016/j.chb.2022.107486

Wei, R. (2020). Ego and cognitive biases in perceptions of media influence. In J. Van Den Bulck (Ed.), *Encyclopedia of media psychology.* New York, NY: Wiley. https://doi.org/10.1002/9781119011071.iemp0228

WHO. (2022, March 2). COVID-19 pandemic triggers 25% increase in prevalence of anxiety and depression worldwide. Retrieved April 2, 2022, from https://www.who.int/news/item/02-03-2022-covid-19-pandemic-triggers-25-increase-in-prevalence-of-anxiety-and-depression-worldwide

Yang, J., & Yu, T. (2021). Others are more vulnerable to fake news than I Am: Third-person effect of COVID-19 fake news on social media users. *Computers in Human Behavior, 125,* 1–10. https://doi.org/10.1016/j.chb.2021.106950.

Zhang, L., Chen, K., Jiang, H., & Zhao, J. (2020). How the health rumor misleads people's perception in a public health emergency: Lessons from a purchase craze during the COVID-19 outbreak in China. *International Journal of Environmental Research and Public Health, 17*(19), 7213. https://doi.org/10.3390/ijerph17197213

7 The Antivax Phenomenon

Trust and Misinformation

Yi-Hui Christine Huang and Jun Li

Introduction

Vaccine hesitancy has been a worldwide phenomenon and noted as a major issue in controlling the COVID-19 pandemic (Lazarus et al., 2022). Misinformation and trust may jointly influence people's anti-vaccine intentions. Vaccine hesitancy can result from both internal and external factors. Internal factors include one's past experience with vaccination, accessibility to vaccines, financial obstacles, and complacency regarding vaccine-preventable diseases (VPDs) (Dubé et al., 2013). External factors originate from people's knowledge about vaccines via their interactions with the social environment; their trust in agencies that produce and administer the vaccination program. These factors are important in shaping individuals' intentions to take jabs (Dubé et al., 2013). In the case of COVID-19, people's trust in pharmaceuticals, medical professionals, and public officials or politicians that promote vaccination may affect their acceptance of vaccines (Allington et al., 2021; Riad et al., 2021). Therefore, the deterioration of institutional trust is very likely to be associated with lower levels of vaccination willingness. Thus, we consider anti-vaccine attitudes to be major negative consequences caused by the spread of COVID-19 misinformation on social media and the distrust in public health authorities during the pandemic. This chapter examines the underlying process of how encounters with misinformation (refer to Chapters 4 and 5) and trust in government shape a respondents' anti-vaccine attitudes in the four studied cities.

Generally, institutional trust can be determined by (1) whether given institutions' performances are satisfactory enough to meet trustors' expectations (Mishler & Roses, 2001; Zimmer, 1979); (2) behaviors of institutional leaders (Zimmer, 1979), as a facet of institutional reputation; (3) negative framing of news about institutions, which may lead to higher levels of discontent from the public (Cappella & Jamieson, 1997); and (4) cultural variables, such as traditional beliefs and civic involvement in the institution (Putnam, 1993; Yang & Tang, 2010). Apart from these factors, institutional trust can be shaped by institutional contexts (e.g., the electoral system and the party system for trust in the government), knowledge and rational assessment of

DOI: 10.4324/9781003355984-7

trustees, propensities of trustors as well as social capital or higher levels of social trust (Barber, 1983; Criado & Herreros, 2007; Kramer, 1999; Nannestad, 2008; Putnam, 1993).

Research (Dubé et al., 2013; Jennings et al., 2021; Schernhammer et al., 2022) underscores the role of institutional trust (government trust in particular) in affecting people's vaccine acceptance, largely because authorities have been responsible for calling on collective action by citizens to comply with preventive measures against the pandemic (Van Oost et al., 2022). When it comes to vaccination as a preventive measure that involves potential health-related risks, institutional trust, including both the trust in the institution's motive and trust in the institution's competence (Jamison et al., 2019; Siegrist et al., 2003; Twyman et al., 2008), is a prominent value for citizen collaboration (Siegrist et al., 2003). In the case of COVID-19 vaccination, such trust can motivate people to participate in collective action and contribute to the establishment of herd immunity despite potential health risks that may be caused by taking jabs (Van Oost et al., 2022). A lower level of institutional trust, on the other hand, may cause people to suspect vaccine information provided by official sources and engender self-interested resistance against preventive measures (Dubé et al., 2013; Jamison et al., 2019; Yaqub et al., 2014). What is worse, distrust in institutions that produce or administer vaccines can even lead to conspiracy theories against state agencies, pharmaceuticals, and/ or health agencies as well as professionals (Van Oost et al., 2022), further discouraging people from taking COVID-19 vaccines.

Misinformation is another shaping factor that may affect people's acceptance of vaccines. As defined in Chapter 1, misinformation refers to misleading information and rumors that among other things have been proved to prevent the public from getting vaccinated (Puri et al., 2020). Also, in Chapter 6, we reported that misinformation triggered negative emotions such as anger, anxiety, fear, and panic (Dubé et al., 2015; Peretti-Watel et al., 2014), which give rise to the affective risks associated with vaccination (Featherstone & Zhang, 2020). Likewise, misinformation can also stir political distrust toward the government and increase cynicism as well as apathy (Cappella & Jamieson, 1997; Kleinnijenhuis et al., 2006; Ognyanova et al., 2020), or fan support for populist leaders (Hooghe, 2018; Ognyanova et al., 2020). This is where misinformation indirectly works on people's attitudes toward the state-administered vaccination. Under the current media environment, social media have become a hotbed for spreading misinformation due to their prevalence. Social media give rise to online communities that attract like-minded people, creating echo chambers that reinforce their opinions and self-select media content (Muric et al., 2021; Puri et al., 2020). This actually facilitates the polarization of vaccine supporters and vaccine opponents both on social media and in daily life.

In short, this chapter examines the negative effect of misinformation and the institutional trust on the anti-vaccine attitudes of respondents in Beijing, Hong Kong, Singapore, and Taipei. We focus on the dimension of "institutional trust" in the broad concept of trust in government because it is a significant sub-type of institutional trust and crucial to immunization programs in the current public health crisis. To better describe the underlying mechanism of how misinformation and institutional trust works we examined five variables—misinformation exposure, sharing, elaboration, negative emotions, and government trust—as independent variables that predict people's anti-vaccine attitudes. By including these key variables, we aimed to reveal the causal chain connecting misinformation, trust in government as well as attitudes toward vaccines.

Government Trust and Anti-Vaccine Attitudes in Four Cities

Government trust has been studied from two approaches: the performance approach and the cultural approach (Mishler & Roses, 2001; Wong et al., 2011). The performance approach refers to the government's perceived performance and reputation (Cappella & Jamieson, 1997; Mishler & Roses, 2001; Zimmer, 1979). Apart from the aforementioned performance-related factors, government trust is also affected by culture (Almond & Verba, 1963; Inglehart, 1999; Yang & Tang, 2010). In the West, the tradition of public participation has been considered a shaping factor for people's trust in the government (Putnam, 1993). The civic engagement in northern Italy, for example, encouraged political deliberation among citizens, consolidating their support for the government (Putnam, 1993).

Asian societies have provided a less fertile soil for civic engagement due to their long history of authoritarian rule and hierarchical structure (Shi, 2014). Government trust in Asian societies, therefore, originates from different cultural sources. To Asian cultures, political trust can be built on the basis of traditional social values, such as strict hierarchies within the society and limited or no open competition among interest groups, while the state in return must take into key consideration the people's collective interests (Shi, 2014). Moreover, traditional family values prevailing in Asian societies such as family conformity and the emphasis on family interests also provide a catalyst for people's favorable opinions of government officials (Zhai, 2018). That being said, research on vaccine acceptance and political trust in the Asian cultural context is needed due to different state-society dynamics across Asian societies. Thus, we have intended to provide an Asian perspective in terms of government trust and attempted to explore how the tradition of political trust and encounter with misinformation can jointly affect people's anti-vaccine attitudes.

Despite the similar influences of culture, past studies have shown differences in government trust among leading Chinese societies. Mainland China is characteristic of high political trust due to satisfactory economic performance, growing global influence, traditional cultural values, and nationalism (Wong et al., 2011). Like Mainland China, Singapore also enjoys a high level of political trust, but cultural values do not play an important role in Singaporeans' government trust (Wong et al., 2011). Different from Mainlanders, Hongkongers' political trust is determined by economic performance and democratic rights rather than cultural values (Wong et al., 2009). Citizens in Taiwan are susceptible to the influence of traditional values, as well as government performances and democratic rights, but a lower level of political trust among Taiwanese has been the norm (Wong et al., 2009).

It is worth noting that the public's attitudes toward vaccines are less polarized in the four societies. The COVID-19 vaccination rates in the four cities have reached more than 80%. Nevertheless, segments of the population still resist the jab. Misinformation and lack of trust in the government are considered to influence people's decisions on vaccination. Studies have shown that people's willingness to get vaccinated in Singapore and Taiwan may be significantly but negatively related to misinformation (Chen et al., 2022; Tan et al., 2022). On the other hand, trust in the government was found to boost people's confidence in vaccination, counteracting the negative impacts of misinformation (Jin et al., 2022; Lau et al., 2022; Tan et al., 2022).

In a nutshell, the sweeping COVID-19 pandemic has posed new challenges to both the government capability and government trust worldwide. Theories have emerged to explain the variation in people's political support during the crisis; while some scholars have stressed the facilitating effect of crisis on people's political support (Schraff, 2021), others have indicated a decline of public confidence in the government after the surge of patriotic sentiments (Davies et al., 2021). Vaccination is a crucial facet of public health management that is influenced by popular support for the government.

Against this backdrop, our investigation into government trust and anti-vaccine attitudes in the four societies contributes to both studies of trust and theories of public health management. The findings have implications for how to tackle the issue of policy compliance in an era of social media.

Findings

Operationally, *government trust* was measured by three questions that tapped respondents' evaluations on their government's efficiency and competitiveness: (1) "The government is efficient at the things they try to do," (2) "The government is equipped with adequate technical skills in epidemic control," and (3) "The government is competent in epidemic prevention." Responses on a 5-point Likert scale (1 = strongly disagree, 5 = strongly agree) were combined into an index of government trust ($M = 3.40$, $SD = 1.08$, $\alpha = .88$).

For *anti-vaccine attitudes*, the dependent variable of this chapter, a number of factors associated with anti-vaccine attitudes were measured by questions that asked respondents to report their opinions about vaccine safety and effectiveness: (1) "People are deceived about the effectiveness of COVID-19 vaccines," (2) "Data about COVID-19 vaccine effectiveness is fabricated," and (3) "People are deceived about COVID-19 vaccine safety" (1 = strongly disagree, 5 = strongly agree). Responses were combined to form an index measuring anti-vaccine attitudes ($M = 2.50$, $SD = 1.10$, $\alpha = .90$).

Demographic Patterns of Anti-Vaccine Attitudes

To determine shaping factors for anti-vaccine attitudes, we conducted a series of independent-sample t-tests to compare the anti-vaccine attitudes of the respondents with different demographic characteristics such as gender and age, misinformation-related behaviors, negative emotions, and government trust in the four studied cities.

How male ($n = 1,978$) and female respondents ($n = 2,116$) felt about vaccines were explored first. No significant difference was found in the overall level of anti-vaccine attitudes between male ($M = 2.50$, $SD = 1.14$) and female respondents ($M = 2.51$, $SD = 1.05$), $t = -0.32$, $p > .05$. Likewise, male ($M = 2.47$, $SD = 1.23$) and female respondents ($M = 2.48$, $SD = 1.13$) did not express divided opinions on whether people are deceived about the effectiveness of COVID-19 vaccines ($t = -0.41$, $p > .05$). Nor did male ($M = 2.45$, $SD = 1.24$) and female respondents ($M = 2.49$, $SD = 1.16$) have significant disagreement on the statement that data about COVID-19 vaccine effectiveness is fabricated ($t = -1.20$, $p > .05$). Male ($M = 2.57$, $SD = 1.27$) and female respondents ($M = 2.54$, $SD = 1.17$) also responded in a similar way whether people are deceived about COVID-19 vaccine safety ($t = 0.70$, $p > .05$). Therefore, gender made no difference in affecting respondents' anti-vaccine attitudes.

People of different ages did not hold divided attitudes toward vaccines, either. Young respondents (i.e., 18–39; $n = 2,051$) and old (i.e., 40–84; $n = 2,042$) reacted to anti-vaccine statements. Both groups showed little difference in these statements; younger respondents ($M = 2.52$, $SD = 1.12$) and older ($M = 2.49$, $SD = 1.07$) had no difference in their overall attitudes ($t = 0.91$, $p > .05$). Meanwhile, no difference was found between younger ($M = 2.47$, $SD = 1.19$) and older respondents ($M = 2.49$, $SD = 1.17$) on their agreement whether people are deceived about the effectiveness of COVID-19 vaccines ($t = -0.55$, $p > .05$). Younger ($M = 2.51$, $SD = 1.22$) and older respondents ($M = 2.44$, $SD = 1.17$) felt similarly about whether data on vaccine effectiveness is fabricated ($t = 1.87$, $p > .05$). They also appeared alike on the statement that "people are deceived about COVID-19 vaccine safety" ($t = 1.14$, $p > .05$).

Misinformation and Anti-Vaccine Attitudes

The results of independent-sample t-tests between encountering misinformation and anti-vaccine attitudes are presented in Table 7.1. We divided misinformation exposure into a low-exposure group ($n = 1,858$) and a high-exposure group ($n = 2,236$; see Chapter 4 for measures used). The cutoff point was the median value of responses. Different attitudes towards vaccines held by people with different levels of misinformation exposure existed.

Table 7.1 Differences in anti-vaccine attitudes between individuals of low and high
level of misinformation exposure

	Low exposure (n = 1,858)	High exposure (n = 2,236)	
	M (SD)	M (SD)	t value
1 People are deceived about the effectiveness of COVID-19 vaccines	2.38 (1.12)	2.56 (1.23)	–4.99***
2 Data about COVID-19 vaccine effectiveness is fabricated	2.30 (1.06)	2.61 (1.28)	–8.44***
3 People are deceived about COVID-19 vaccine safety	2.42 (1.10)	2.67 (1.30)	–6.64***
Combined index	2.37 (0.99)	2.61 (1.17)	–7.32***

Note: The items were rated from 1 to 5, where 1 = strongly disagree and 5 = strongly agree;
***p < .001.

In general, respondents with low exposure to misinformation (M = 2.37, SD = .99) significantly had less anti-vaccine attitudes than did people with high exposure (M = 2.61, SD = 1.17), t = –7.32, p < .001. Specifically, respondents of low exposure to misinformation (M = 2.38, SD = 1.12) showed significantly less doubts about the effectiveness of vaccines than did those of high exposure to misinformation (M = 2.56, SD = 1.23), t = –4.99, p < .001. Respondents of low exposure to misinformation (M = 2.30, SD = 1.06) were also less suspicious about the validity of vaccine effectiveness data than were respondents of high exposure (M = 2.61, SD = 1.28). The difference was significant (t = –8.44, p < .001). Furthermore, respondents of low exposure (M = 2.42, SD = 1.10) were less likely to believe that people are deceived about the vaccine safety than were people of high exposure (M = 2.67, SD = 1.30), t = –6.64, p < .001.

Table 7.2 presents how misinformation sharing was related to anti-vaccine attitudes. We categorized 2,337 respondents as "low sharing," and 1,757 respondents as "high sharing" (Chapter 5 details the measure). People with low misinformation sharing (M = 2.33, SD = 1.00) opposed the COVID-19 vaccines significantly less compared to those with high misinformation sharing (M = 2.72, SD = 1.17), t = –11.09, p < .001. The low misinformation sharing group (M = 2.32, SD = 1.11) agreed less that people are deceived about vaccine effectiveness, compared to those with high misinformation sharing (M = 2.68, SD = 1.24), t = –9.77, p < .001. Also, respondents with low misinformation sharing showed less doubt about the validity of vaccine effectiveness data (M = 2.27, SD = 1.07), t = –12.53, p < .001, and vaccine safety (M = 2.42, SD = 1.13), t = –8.18, p < .001

Table 7.3 shows anti-vaccine attitudes by the high misinformation elaboration group (n = 1,979) and the low misinformation elaboration group (n = 2,115). To assess the elaboration of COVID-19 misinformation, four

Table 7.2 Differences in anti-vaccine attitudes during the COVID-19 pandemic between individuals of low and high level of sharing

	Low sharing (n = 2,337)	High sharing (n = 1,757)	
	M (SD)	M (SD)	t value
1 People are deceived about the effectiveness of COVID-19 vaccines	2.32 (1.11)	2.68 (1.24)	−9.77***
2 Data about COVID-19 vaccine effectiveness is fabricated	2.27 (1.07)	2.74 (1.30)	−12.53***
3 People are deceived about COVID-19 vaccine safety	2.42 (1.13)	2.74 (1.31)	−8.18***
Combined index	2.33 (1.00)	2.72 (1.17)	−11.09***

Note: The items were rated from 1 to 5, where 1 = strongly disagree and 5 = strongly agree; ***p < .001.

Table 7.3 Differences in anti-vaccine attitudes between individuals of low and high level of elaboration

	Low elaboration (n = 2,115)	High elaboration (n = 1,979)	
	M (SD)	M (SD)	t value
1 People are deceived about the effectiveness of COVID-19 vaccines	2.52 (1.03)	2.43 (1.32)	2.19*
2 Data about COVID-19 vaccine effectiveness is fabricated	2.52 (1.06)	2.42 (1.33)	2.56*
3 People are deceived about COVID-19 vaccine safety	2.63 (1.08)	2.48 (1.35)	3.99***
Combined index	2.56 (.94)	2.45 (1.24)	3.18**

Note: The items were rated from 1 to 5, where 1 = strongly disagree and 5 = strongly agree; *p < .05, **p < .01, ***p < .001.

statements were used on a five-point Likert scale (1 = "strongly disagree" and 5 = "strongly agree"): After exposure to misinformation about COVID-19, (1) I have thought about the issue of misinformation; (2) I have thought about its impact on the pandemic; (3) I have thought about consequences of misinformation; and (4) I often think about how COVID-19 misinformation relates to other COVID-19 information I know. The items were averaged to form a composite measure (M = 3.71, SD = .76, α = .86).

Interestingly, the high misinformation elaboration (M = 2.45, SD = 1.24) group held lower anti-vaccine attitudes (t = 3.18, p < .01). People with high misinformation elaboration (M = 2.43, SD = 1.32) doubted less the effectiveness of COVID-19 vaccines than those with low misinformation elaboration

($M = 2.52$, $SD = 1.03$), $t = 2.19$, $p < .05$. The high misinformation elaboration group ($M = 2.42$, $SD = 1.33$) also did not question the validity of vaccine effectiveness data as fabricated, compared to the low misinformation elaboration group ($M = 2.52$, $SD = 1.06$), $t = 2.56$, $p < .05$. In addition, people with high misinformation elaboration ($M = 2.48$, $SD = 1.35$) agreed less that people are deceived about COVID-19 vaccine safety ($t = 3.99$, $p < .001$).

Negative Emotions and Anti-Vaccine Attitudes

In the absence of scientific knowledge, negative emotions may work as a source of public resistance against vaccines (Chou & Budenz, 2020; Dubé et al., 2013). With the median value of responses as the cutoff point, we categorized the 4,049 respondents into groups of low negative emotions ($n = 1,678$) and high negative emotions ($n = 2,416$) to explore whether people with different levels of negative emotions would have different anti-vaccine attitudes. The measure of emotions can be found in Chapter 6.

As results in Table 7.4 present, the difference in anti-vaccine attitudes (both the index and individual items) between low negative emotions ($M = 2.49$, $SD = .90$) and high negative emotions ($M = 2.51$, $SD = 1.21$) was not significant ($t = -0.45$, $p > .05$). These results suggest that public's anti-vaccine attitudes were not affected by levels of negative emotions.

Government Trust and Anti-Vaccine Attitudes

To find out if people's confidence in the government under the pandemic can affect their acceptance of COVID-19 vaccines, we categorized respondents by the median value as the cutoff point into two groups: the group of low government trust ($n = 2,196$) and high government trust ($n = 1,898$).

Table 7.4 Differences in anti-vaccine attitudes between individuals of low and high level of negative emotions

	Low negative emotions ($n = 1,678$)	High negative emotions ($n = 2,416$)	
	M (SD)	M (SD)	t value
1 People are deceived about the effectiveness of COVID-19 vaccines	2.44 (1.00)	2.50 (1.29)	−1.60
2 Data about COVID-19 vaccine effectiveness is fabricated	2.47 (1.00)	2.48 (1.31)	−.28
3 People are deceived about COVID-19 vaccine safety	2.57 (1.02)	2.55 (1.39)	.62
Combined index	2.49 (.90)	2.51 (1.21)	−.45

Note: The items were rated from 1 to 5, where 1 = strongly disagree and 5 = strongly agree.

Table 7.5 Differences in anti-vaccine attitudes between individuals of low and high level of government trust

	Low trust (n = 2,196)	High trust (n = 1,898)	
	M (SD)	M (SD)	t value
1 People are deceived about the effectiveness of COVID-19 vaccines	2.46 (1.01)	2.49 (1.31)	–.61
2 Data about COVID-19 vaccine effectiveness is fabricated	2.53 (1.00)	2.43 (1.34)	2.68**
3 People are deceived about COVID-19 vaccine safety	2.64 (1.00)	2.49 (1.38)	4.11***
Combined index	2.54 (.89)	2.47 (1.25)	2.28*

Note: The items were rated from 1 to 5, where 1 = strongly disagree and 5 = strongly agree.

As indicated by Table 7.5, the group of low government trust ($M = 2.54$, $SD = .89$) resisted COVID-19 vaccines more than did the group of high government trust ($M = 2.47$, $SD = 1.25$). The difference was significant ($t = 2.28$, $p < .05$). To be specific, people of low government trust ($M = 2.53$, $SD = 1.00$) felt more strongly that data about COVID-19 vaccine effectiveness is fabricated, compared to people of high government trust ($M = 2.43$, $SD = 1.34$), $t = 2.68$, $p < .01$. Likewise, those of low government trust ($M = 2.64$, $SD = 1.00$) had more concerns that people are deceived about COVID-19 vaccine safety than did high government trust ($M = 2.49$, $SD = 1.38$), $t = 4.11$, $p < .001$. However, people of low government trust ($M = 2.46$, $SD = 1.01$) did not differ from people of high government trust ($M = 2.49$, $SD = 1.31$) in doubting the effectiveness of COVID-19 vaccines ($t = -0.61$, $p > .05$).

Cross-City Differences in Anti-Vaccine Attitudes

Table 7.6 shows results of differences in anti-vaccine attitude among residents in Beijing ($n = 1,033$), Hong Kong ($n = 1,017$), Taipei ($n = 1,019$), and Singapore ($n = 1,025$). Respondents in Beijing ($M = 2.10$, $SD = 1.24$) and Taipei ($M = 2.32$, $SD = .97$) reported lower levels of anti-vaccine attitudes than did their counterparts in Hong Kong ($M = 2.50$, $SD = .97$) and Singapore ($M = 3.09$, $SD = 0.92$), $F(3, 4090) = 172.42$, $p < .001$. Respondents from Beijing ($M = 2.07$, $SD = 1.29$) doubted vaccine effectiveness less than did people in Hong Kong ($M = 2.44$, $SD = 1.01$), Taipei ($M = 2.17$, $SD = 1.03$), and Singapore ($M = 3.23$, $SD = 1.01$), $F(3, 4090) = 237.90$, $p < .001$. People in Beijing ($M = 2.13$, $SD = 1.35$) also had fewer concerns that data for vaccine effectiveness is fabricated than did their counterparts in Hong Kong ($M = 2.47$, $SD = 1.08$), Taipei ($M = 2.37$, $SD = 1.10$), and Singapore ($M = 2.92$, $SD = 1.09$), $F(3, 4090) = 85.11$, $p < .001$. Similarly, respondents in Beijing ($M = 2.10$, $SD = 1.33$) questioned vaccine safety less in comparison to people from Hong Kong ($M = 2.60$, $SD = 1.11$), Taipei ($M = 2.41$, $SD = 1.06$), and Singapore ($M = 3.11$, $SD=1.12$), $F(3, 4090) = 135.21$, $p < .001$.

Table 7.6 Differences in anti-vaccine attitudes across Beijing, Hong Kong, Taipei, and Singapore

	Beijing (n = 1,033)	Hong Kong (n = 1,017)	Taipei (n = 1,019)	Singapore (n = 1,025)	Total	F value
1 People are deceived about the effectiveness of COVID-19 vaccines	2.07 (1.29)	2.44 (1.01)	2.17 (1.03)	3.23 (1.01)	2.48 (1.18)	237.90***
2 Data about COVID-19 vaccine effectiveness is fabricated	2.13 (1.35)	2.47 (1.08)	2.37 (1.10)	2.92 (1.09)	2.47 (1.20)	85.11***
3 People are deceived about COVID-19 vaccine safety	2.10 (1.33)	2.60 (1.11)	2.41 (1.06)	3.11 (1.12)	2.56 (1.22)	135.21***
Combined index	2.10 (1.24)	2.50 (.97)	2.32 (.97)	3.09 (.92)	2.50 (1.10)	172.42***

Note: The items were rated from 1 to 5, where 1 = strongly disagree and 5 = strongly agree; ***$p < .001$.

Predictors of Anti-Vaccine Attitudes

Next, to identify the most significant predictors of anti-vaccine attitudes, we conducted a hierarchical regression on the attitudes with demographic factors, misinformation-related behaviors, negative emotions, and government trust as the predictors. Results are summarized in Table 7.7.

With the influence of key demographics (i.e., gender, age, education, and city) being controlled, all the misinformation-related behaviors, including misinformation exposure ($\beta = .32$, $p < .001$), misinformation sharing ($\beta = .15$, $p < .001$), and misinformation elaboration ($\beta = -.08$, $p < .001$) turned out to be significantly related to anti-vaccine attitudes. That is, higher levels of misinformation exposure and sharing led to stronger anti-vaccine attitudes, while misinformation elaboration helped to decrease people's resistance against vaccines. Such differences in effects may be caused by levels of cognitive activities required for people to perform misinformation-related behaviors. When people were engaged in misinformation exposure and sharing, they were possibly in a state of "cognitive overload," which usually takes place when people are overwhelmed by the flux of information on social media, leaving limited cognitive resources at their disposal (Islam et al., 2020). Also, refer to Chapter 9 for our own analyses on the issue.

The issue of "cognitive overload" gives rise to people's social media fatigue and furthermore hinders people from verifying online information they have

Table 7.7 Hierarchical regression analysis predicting anti-vaccine attitudes

Predictors	Anti-vaccine attitudes
Block 1: Demographics	
Age	.05**
Gender (Male = 1)	−.02
Education	−.03*
City (Beijing = 1)	−.30***
Adjusted R^2	4.5%
Block 2: Misinformation exposure	
Misinformation exposure	.32***
Incremental adjusted R^2	11.6%
Block 3: Misinformation sharing	
Misinformation sharing	.15***
Incremental adjusted R^2	1.6%
Block 4: Elaboration of misinformation	
Elaboration	−.08***
Incremental adjusted R^2	0.4%
Block 5: Negative emotions	
Negative emotions	.04*
Incremental adjusted R^2	0%
Block 6: Government trust	
Government trust	−.04**
Incremental adjusted R^2	0.2%
Total adjusted R^2	18.3%

Note: N = 4,093; **p < .01, ***p < .001; the age entry has one missing value.

viewed or shared (Islam et al., 2020). However, when people move into the phase of "misinformation elaboration," they are motivated to allocate cognitive resources and evaluate the misinformation they are exposed to, which cancels potential detriments to the public health caused by misinformation (Islam et al., 2020). That is to say, "misinformation elaboration" may require a different type of cognitive-information processing from "misinformation exposure" and "misinformation sharing," and therefore their effects differ from encounters with misinformation.

Negative emotions were a significant predictor of anti-vaccine attitudes (β = .04, p < .05). Consistent with past research (Jin et al., 2022), government trust (β = −.04, p < .01) plays a moderately significant role in diluting public resistance against vaccines, meaning that more trust in the government can enhance people's acceptance of COVID-19 vaccines. As government efforts are still required for the promotion of vaccines among the general public, especially those of vulnerable communities, this result indicates the importance of timely communications and guidelines from the government to increase people's willingness to get vaccinated.

Lastly, it is worth noting that city of residence (β = −.21, p < .001) turned out to be a significant predictor of anti-vaccine attitudes. Respondents in Beijing were more willing to take jabs, compared with people from the other three societies. The results point to the role of contextual factors in shaping peoples' vaccine attitudes.

Summary of Key Findings

With regard to attitudes, results of this chapter illustrate the major attitudinal differences toward vaccines among respondents in the four Chinese societies. Multivariate analyses identified a number of contributing factors (e.g., misinformation-related behaviors, negative emotions, and their trust in the government) that explain the differences. The key findings are recaptured as follows:

- There is no gender or age difference in anti-vaccine attitudes. Only city of residence made a difference. Respondents in Beijing had the highest level of trust in vaccines, followed by people in Taipei. Singaporeans had the lowest level of trust in vaccines.
- Respondents of high misinformation exposure distrusted vaccines significantly more than did low-exposure respondents. Likewise, respondents of high misinformation sharing distrusted vaccines significantly more than did low-sharing respondents.
- However, respondents of high misinformation elaboration trusted significantly more in vaccines than did low-elaboration respondents. So did those with high levels of trust in government.
- Accordingly, exposure to and sharing of misinformation were positively related (i.e., enhancing) to anti-vaccine attitudes while elaboration and government trust were negatively related to (i.e., decreasing) the negative attitudes. Given the highest level of public trust in the Chinese government, it is not surprising that residents in Beijing were found to trust vaccines more than did people from the other three societies.

Qualitative Findings

Trust: The Key for Vaccination

Observations and personal accounts by participants in the focus groups underscore the role of trust in the government in mass vaccination campaigns. Lower government trust may lead to citizens questioning the government's motivations to call on collective action by citizens to get vaccinated as a preventive measure. A 41-year-old male participant James in Hong Kong shared his observation of distrust of the government's COVID policy in Hong Kong, especially its vaccine campaign. He said,

> the government is really doing everything it can to get everyone vaccinated like it has tasks to accomplish, and the health promotion of vaccines is not for the benefit of citizens. According to them, if one gets

sick, the cause would be not being vaccinated, and when something happens to someone, they said that it's nothing to do with the vaccines.

Even participants who indicated that they trusted the government did not give the government a blank check. The 40-year-old male participant from Singapore, Michael, still believed that "we can feel that the government is working on the COVID-19 pandemic, but I don't think they always push what's best for the people."

Moreover, lower government trust may lead citizens to doubt the authenticity of data concerning COVID-19 vaccines from health authorities and even health professionals in mass media, lowering confidence in the safety and efficacy of COVID-19 vaccines. Participants said they intensively sought advice from health professionals they knew and health experiences from friends around them. A 22-year-old female student from Singapore, Camila, said that before deciding whether to take vaccines, one would "need more information and what the side effects may be." Another female participant Emily also from Singapore, who got vaccinated herself, remained hesitant to let her children take the shots. She explained why:

> I'm still not comfortable yet, because I feel that even with the information I read, I still don't get assurance that the one reading is really the whole picture. So, I'm not going to vaccinate my kid so soon, I am not going to jump on the bandwagon to vaccinate my child. Maybe give it another six months and wait until I can chat with the pediatrician.

Unlike Emily, who may still go to the pediatrician for recommendations, a 54-year-old male engineer in Singapore Jackson did not seek vaccine-related information himself. He read messages forwarded by friends and advice from health authorities and medical professionals in the media. Whenever the two accounts conflicted, he said, he preferred to follow friends' personal experiences on vaccination. "I don't have to go and search," he explained.

> I see what was forwarded many times. So normally, I will read, then there's also media, the ones who speak normally, you can see they are doctors, professors from the university, specialists from doing some research. So, I don't think they're as bad as our government. They are also equally qualified. It's just that they may be spreading... I don't know whether a specialist will spread negative news. I do not know, but I take it as just a piece of general information. Until today, I really do not know which are true facts, and which are not true facts. I don't 100% believe what government says is correct because I see friends with vaccination, a friend's father with vaccination also passed away because of COVID. So, to me now, I don't know which is real and which is untrue, but at least I know one thing. The personal immune system is the most important. That's all I know.

A younger female Singaporean fashion designer, Abigail, shared some thoughts similar to Jackson's. In her words,

> Yeah, I didn't really search online, but I would consult my friends who already got a vaccination. So, they will tell me about the different vaccination and what will happen to you. So, from there, I will make the judgment and decide what to do with it.

Misinformation Has Consequences

If trust in government is a deciding factor in taking the vaccine shot, exposure to COVID-19 misinformation is another factor in weighing the pros and cons of shots. According to the participants, encountering misinformation contributed to developing anti-vaccine attitudes and their decisions. Summarizing from the discussions, they revealed that they encountered several types of such misinformation, including about the development speed of the vaccines, their efficacy and safety. Participants were against COVID-19 vaccines if they believe the vaccines were unsafe because of their hasty development. Such misinformation might further relate to conspiracy, for example, if they believed the government lied about possible side effects of vaccines.

The fashion designer, Abigail, in Singapore, said she believed rumors circulating about the safety of vaccines available in Singapore. According to her account,

> For me, I think they were true. Because I don't really know whether this vaccine is effective or not. [It's still] the initial stage of the vaccine. Some people say that the government is coming up with this vaccine, but there are not enough numbers to prove its effectiveness. So, they're trying out on the seniors first, so they are somehow the first batch of the Guinea pigs to test out this COVID vaccine. That's why the first project is only rolled out to the senior batch, so they are the first batch. The rumors are telling seniors not to fall for the trap. Don't take the vaccine.

Therefore, she told her parents not to get vaccinated: "I told my parents, don't jab first, wait for everyone to jab first. They actually listened and waited a while."

Another 53-year-old male participant Sebastian in Singapore expressed the same concern, feeling that citizens who participated in the vaccine program were being treated like lab animals for experiments. He said,

> I think everyone has the same concern. Actually, whether we are not Guinea pigs for this vaccine is to be questioned. By right, all vaccines should be tested on animals to make sure they're effective. We want one dose for all, not keep asking you to take it every year like a flu vaccine. So, now you see a two-in-one vaccine for the COVID new variant is also not tested yet.

Participants were also against COVID-19 vaccines if they thought that the vaccines might be ineffective or not work for everyone. A 26-year-old female participant Ms. Chen in Beijing explained her thoughts on the relationship between vaccine and immunology. In her own words,

> I think the virus is always mutating. Thus, the vaccine cannot guarantee its effectiveness. For those previous variants, it relies on the individual's immunity too. Moreover, the government said that a good number of people are not recommended for vaccination, patients with hypertension, for instance. Then they said that even patients with hypertension could get it. You see, I think we better evaluate the individual situations with care. To me, improving immunity is the best policy, and it would be a safer guard.

A 58-year-old female participant Ms. Chuang in Taipei did not trust the vaccine's efficacy because, as she put it, "it's too new." She continued,

> The original vaccine is ineffective for the current variants. I don't think that the fourth dose will work. I didn't have much side effect for the first two doses. However, when it came to the third dose, I was not feeling well after the vaccination. It's too new. I went to the doctor, and they don't know why because these are all new.

Almost all of the participants were against COVID-19 vaccines due to other concerns. For instance, they believed that the vaccines might not be safe because they might modify DNA, contain the pathogenic virus, or induce severe side effects. Ms. Zhu, a 41-year-old female participant who works in a state-run company in Beijing, was among the few in Beijing who did not get the vaccine. She said she heard about the side effects of vaccines on boosting the development of cancer and other severe diseases. She explained,

> I've not been vaccinated because I was pregnant last year, so they didn't ask me to take the shot. I heard about the side effects of the vaccine on cancer, my friend told me that the vaccine would stimulate cancer cells. Many people get cancer and need to go to the hospital, and the doctors say that the development of cancers in those people is accelerated because of vaccines. Not only the doctors from oncology-specialized hospitals said so, but the doctors from other hospitals said the same thing. Doctors in Beijing and other cities said so.

Some participants distrusted the vaccine's safety because they had doubts about how the vaccine was developed. Thus, they remained uncertain about its use and delayed getting vaccinated because they feared latent side effects. A 52-year-old Taipei participant Ms. Lo, who works at a hotel reception, indicated that she did not feel comfortable with the idea of healthy people taking the vaccine, which is "extracted from the virus." A younger male student in Hong Kong Elijah said he preferred not to get vaccinated due to the fear that it would modify his DNA. He continued,

> It seems that there's research that found out the Pfizer-BioNTech COVID-19 vaccine will disrupt your genetic sequence. I'm not sure about the possibility of having a baby with a deficiency in the future because of it. So, I have concerns about getting the vaccination.

Conclusion and Insights

Analyses in this chapter offer new insights concerning how to limit or control the harmful effects of misinformation on the public's negative attitudes toward COVID-19 vaccines. Because elaboration of misinformation enhances trust in vaccine effectiveness and safety, the government can plan public education programs to make citizens reflect on the detriments of misinformation in addition to consider regulating the spread of misinformation in society.

Moreover, efforts should be made to enhance institutional trust in encouraging people to take vaccines during a public health crisis. As the vaccination programs around the world are initiated by the government, strengthening people's confidence in the government can enhance their evaluation on the effectiveness of vaccines, thus boosting positive attitudes to vaccination. Thus, it is highly advisable for the government to establish channels between public officials and citizens, demonstrating higher levels of reliability and competence.

To sum up, this chapter focused on examining the harmful effects of misinformation on anti-vaccine attitudes in Beijing, Hong Kong, Taipei, and Singapore. We derive new findings from the analyses and provided evidence-based insightful recommendations to reduce public's resistance to vaccination during the COVID-19 pandemic. The next chapter will further examine the adverse effects of COVID-19 misinformation on the respondents' cognitive outcomes (beliefs about misinformation and knowledge about the pandemic).

References

Allington, D., McAndrew, S., Moxham-Hall, V., & Duffy, B. (2021). Coronavirus conspiracy suspicions, general vaccine attitudes, trust, and coronavirus information source as predictors of vaccine hesitancy among UK residents during the COVID-19 pandemic. *Psychological Medicine*, 1–12. https://doi.org/10.1017/S0033291721001434

Almond, G., & Verba, S. (1963). *The civic culture*. Princeton: Princeton University Press.

Barber, B. (1983). *The logic and limits of trust*. New Brunswick: Rutgers University Press.

Cappella, J. N., & Jamieson, K. H. (1997). *Spiral of cynicism: The press and the public good*. Oxford: Oxford University Press.

Chen, Y.-P., Chen, Y.-Y., Yang, K.-C., Lai, F., Huang, C.-H., Chen, Y.-N., & Tu, Y.-C. (2022). The prevalence and impact of fake news on COVID-19 vaccination in Taiwan: Retrospective study of digital media. *Journal of Medical Internet Research, 24*(4), e36830. https://doi.org/10.2196/36830

Chou, W.-Y. S., & Budenz, A. (2020). Considering emotion in COVID-19 vaccine communication: Addressing vaccine hesitancy and fostering vaccine confidence. *Health Communication, 35*(14), 1718–1722. https://doi.org/10.1080/10410236.2020.1838096

Criado, H., & Herreros, F. (2007). Political support: Taking into account the institutional context. *Comparative Political Studies, 40*(12), 1511–1532. https://doi.org/10.1177/0010414006292117

Davies, B., Lalot, F., Peitz, L., Heering, M. S., Ozkececi, H., Babaian, J., ... Abrams, D. (2021). Changes in political trust in Britain during the COVID-19 pandemic in 2020: Integrated public opinion evidence and implications. *Humanities and Social Sciences Communications, 8*(1), 1–9. https://doi.org/10.1057/s41599-021-00850-6

Dubé, E., Laberge, C., Guay, M., Bramadat, P., Roy, R., & Bettinger, J. A. (2013). Vaccine hesitancy: An overview. *Human Vaccines & Immunotherapeutics, 9*(8), 1763–1773. https://doi.org/10.4161/hv.24657

Dubé, E., Vivion, M., & MacDonald, N. E. (2015). Vaccine hesitancy, vaccine refusal and the anti-vaccine movement: Influence, impact and implications. *Expert Review of Vaccines, 14*(1), 99–117. https://doi.org/10.1586/14760584.2015.964212

Featherstone, J. D., & Zhang, J. (2020). Feeling angry: The effects of vaccine misinformation and refutational messages on negative emotions and vaccination attitude. *Journal of Health Communication, 25*(9), 692–702. https://doi.org/10.1080/10810730.2020.1838671

Hooghe, M. (2018). Trust and elections. In E. M. Uslaner (Ed.), *The Oxford handbook of social and political trust* (pp. 617–631). Oxford: Oxford University Press.

Inglehart, R. (1999). Trust, well-being and democracy. In M. Warren (Ed.), *Democracy & trust* (pp. 88–120). Cambridge: Cambridge University Press.

Islam, A. K. M. N., Laato, S., Talukder, S., & Sutinen, E. (2020). Misinformation sharing and social media fatigue during COVID-19: An affordance and cognitive load perspective. *Technological Forecasting and Social Change, 159*, 120201. https://doi.org/10.1016/j.techfore.2020.120201

Jamison, A. M., Quinn, S. C., & Freimuth, V. S. (2019). "You don't trust a government vaccine": Narratives of institutional trust and influenza vaccination among African American and white adults. *Social Science & Medicine, 221*, 87–94. https://doi.org/10.1016/j.socscimed.2018.12.020

Jennings, W., Stoker, G., Bunting, H., Valgarðsson, V. O., Gaskell, J., Devine, D., ... Mills, M. C. (2021). Lack of trust, conspiracy beliefs, and social media use predict COVID-19 vaccine hesitancy. *Vaccines, 9*(6), 593. https://doi.org/10.3390/vaccines9060593

Jin, J., Guo, J., & Wei, R. (2022). Examining the impact of exposure to COVID_19 misinformation on vaccine hesitancy among Beijing Residents. *Communication & Society, 63*, 239–267.

Kleinnijenhuis, J., Van Hoof, A. M., & Oegema, D. (2006). Negative news and the sleeper effect of distrust. *Harvard International Journal of Press/Politics, 11*(2), 86–104. https://doi.org/10.1177/1081180X06286417

Kramer, R. M. (1999). Trust and distrust in organizations: Emerging perspectives, enduring questions. *Annual Review of Psychology, 50*, 569–598. https://doi.org/10.1146/annurev.psych.50.1.569

Lau, B. H. P., Yuen, S. W. H., Yue, R. P. H., & Grépin, K. A. (2022). Understanding the societal factors of vaccine acceptance and hesitancy: Evidence from Hong Kong. *Public Health, 207*, 39–45. https://doi.org/10.1016/j.puhe.2022.03.013

Lazarus, J. V., Wyka, K., White, T. M., Picchio, C. A., Rabin, K., Ratzan, S. C., … El-Mohandes, A. (2022). Revisiting COVID-19 vaccine hesitancy around the world using data from 23 countries in 2021. *Nature Communications, 13*(1), 1–14. https://doi.org/10.1038/s41467-022-31441-x

Mishler, W., & Rose, R. (2001). What are the origins of political trust? Testing institutional and cultural theories in post-communist societies. *Comparative Political Studies, 34*(1), 30–62. https://doi.org/10.1177/0010414001034001002

Muric, G., Wu, Y., & Ferrara, E. (2021). COVID-19 vaccine hesitancy on social media: Building a public Twitter data set of anti-vaccine content, vaccine misinformation, and conspiracies. *JMIR Public Health and Surveillance, 7*(11), e30642. https://doi.org/10.2196/30642

Nannestad, P. (2008). What have we learned about generalized trust, if anything? *Annual Review of Political Science, 11*, 413–436. https://doi.org/10.1146/annurev.polisci.11.060606.135412

Ognyanova, K., Lazer, D., Robertson, R. E., & Wilson, C. (2020). Misinformation in action: Fake news exposure is linked to lower trust in media, higher trust in government when your side is in power. *Harvard Kennedy School Misinformation Review, 1*(4), 1–19. https://doi.org/10.37016/mr-2020-024

Peretti-Watel, P., Raude, J., Sagaon-Teyssier, L., Constant, A., Verger, P., & Beck, F. (2014). Attitudes toward vaccination and the H1N1 vaccine: Poor people's unfounded fears or legitimate concerns of the elite? *Social Science & Medicine, 109*, 10–18. https://doi.org/10.1016/j.socscimed.2014.02.035

Puri, N., Coomes, E. A., Haghbayan, H., & Gunaratne, K. (2020). Social media and vaccine hesitancy: New updates for the era of COVID-19 and globalized infectious diseases. *Human Vaccines & Immunotherapeutics, 16*(11), 2586–2593. https://doi.org/10.1080/21645515.2020.1780846

Putnam, R. D. (1993). *Making democracy work*. Princeton: Princeton University Press.

Riad, A., Abdulqader, H., Morgado, M., Domnori, S., Koščík, M., Mendes, J. J., … IADS-SCORE. (2021). Global prevalence and drivers of dental students' COVID-19 vaccine hesitancy. *Vaccines, 9*(6), 566. https://doi.org/10.3390/vaccines9060566

Schernhammer, E., Weitzer, J., Laubichler, M. D., Birmann, B. M., Bertau, M., Zenk, L., … Steiner, G. (2022). Correlates of COVID-19 vaccine hesitancy in Austria: Trust and the government. *Journal of Public Health, 44*(1), e106–e116. https://doi.org/10.1093/pubmed/fdab122

Schraff, D. (2021). Political trust during the Covid-19 pandemic: Rally around the flag or lockdown effects? *European Journal of Political Research, 60*(4), 1007–1017. https://doi.org/10.1111/1475-6765.12425

Shi, T. (2014).*The cultural logic of politics in mainland China and Taiwan*. North Carolina: Cambridge University Press.

Siegrist, M., Earle, T. C., & Gutscher, H. (2003). Test of a trust and confidence model in the applied context of electromagnetic field (EMF) risks. *Risk Analysis: An International Journal, 23*(4), 705–716. https://doi.org/10.1111/1539-6924.00349

Tan, M., Straughan, P. T., & Cheong, G. (2022). Information trust and COVID-19 vaccine hesitancy amongst middle-aged and older adults in Singapore: A latent class analysis Approach. *Social Science & Medicine, 296*, 114767. https://doi.org/10.1016/j.socscimed.2022.114767

Twyman, M., Harvey, N., & Harries, C. (2008). Trust in motives, trust in competence: Separate factors determining the effectiveness of risk communication. *Judgment and Decision Making, 3*(1), 111. https://sjdm.org/~baron/journal/bb10.pdf

Van Oost, P., Yzerbyt, V., Schmitz, M., Vansteenkiste, M., Luminet, O., Morbée, S., … Klein, O. (2022). The relation between conspiracism, government trust, and COVID-19 vaccination intentions: The key role of motivation. *Social Science & Medicine, 301*, 114926. https://doi.org/10.1016/j.socscimed.2022.114926

Wong, T. K., Wan, P., & Hsiao, H.-H. M. (2011). The bases of political trust in six Asian societies: Institutional and cultural explanations compared. *International Political Science Review, 32*(3), 263–281. https://doi.org/10.1177/0192512110378657

Wong, T. K.-Y., Hsiao, H.-H. M., & Wan, P.-S. (2009). Comparing political trust in Hong Kong and Taiwan: Levels, determinants, and implications. *Japanese Journal of Political Science, 10*(2), 147–174. https://doi.org/10.1017/S146810990900351X

Yang, Q., & Tang, W. (2010). Exploring the sources of institutional trust in China: Culture, mobilization, or performance? *Asian Politics & Policy, 2*(3), 415–436. https://doi.org/10.1111/j.1943-0787.2010.01201.x

Yaqub, O., Castle-Clarke, S., Sevdalis, N., & Chataway, J. (2014). Attitudes to vaccination: A critical review. *Social Science & Medicine, 112*, 1–11. https://doi.org/10.1016/j.socscimed.2014.04.018

Zhai, Y. (2018). Traditional values and political trust in China. *Journal of Asian and African Studies, 53*(3), 350–365. https://doi.org/10.1177/0021909616684860

Zimmer, T. A. (1979). The impact of Watergate on the public's trust in people and confidence in the mass media. *Social Science Quarterly, 59*(4), 743–751. http://www.jstor.org/stable/4286047

8 The Cognitive Outcomes of Misinformation

Misbeliefs and Knowledge

Ran Wei and Jing Guo

Introduction

The consequences of widespread misinformation about COVID-19 are far-reaching. The previous two chapters (i.e., Chapters 6 and 7) discussed the detrimental effects of misinformation exposure on individuals' emotional states, risk perceptions, and attitudes toward vaccines in the four cities. Research (Chong et al., 2021; Chou et al., 2020; Lee et al., 2020) also shows that misinformation may harm people's cognitive capacities, such as forming beliefs and acquiring knowledge about the virus. Misbeliefs are fundamentally false perceptions. As McKinley and Lauby (2021) argued, misinformation circulating on social media, such as "COVID-19 vaccines will affect fertility" or "COVID-19 vaccines will alter human DNA," will likely make people develop false beliefs about the efficacy and negative effects of vaccines. Misinformation about channels of COVID-19 transmission and side effects of vaccines has led to vaccine hesitancy in the Asian cities of our study (in Hong Kong in particular, see Wei et al., 2022) because it has caused confusion and misunderstanding about COVID-19 and the pandemic among members of the public.

Moreover, repeated contact with false claims may make people accept them as true (Pluviano et al., 2017). The prevalence of the wide-spreading infodemic on social media platforms during the pandemic in Asia (refer to Chapters 2 and 3) gives rise to a question about what harms COVID-19 misinformation may inflict on the citizens' cognitive abilities in comprehending and acquiring knowledge about the pandemic. To address this question, we examine in this chapter the links between encounters with COVID-19 misinformation (e.g., exposure, sharing, and elaboration) and two cognitive outcome variables: misbeliefs (e.g., accepting misinformation as true) and knowledge acquired about the coronavirus.

Misbeliefs and Knowledge about COVID-19

According to the Health Belief Model (HBM), people develop their own beliefs as perceptions about a disease (e.g., cancer, HIV, and COVID-19). Such beliefs can be multi-dimensional. In the present study, we focus on two

DOI: 10.4324/9781003355984-8

inverse cognitive outcomes in the context of infodemic: misbeliefs about COVID-19 misinformation and de-learning as a result of encountering the misinformation. Our focus is based on the premise that misinformation is seemingly true but factually incorrect. If a person thinks that a piece of debunked misinformation like "COVID-19 vaccines will alter human DNA" or "Drinking bleach can kill COVID-19 virus" to be likely or definitely true, the person is considered to have misbeliefs. In a similar vein, half-truths about COVID-19 that are catchy and attractive (refer to Chapter 2), may hinder the knowledge people acquire about the disease by causing confusion or doubts about factually correct knowledge, resulting in learning less about the disease, what Wei et al. (2022) called a "de-learning" effect (p. 245).

Evidence accumulating in the literature indicates a link between misbeliefs and knowledge and exposure to COVID-19 misinformation on social media (Pennycook et al., 2020; Wei et al., 2022) in addition to demographics (Gerosa et al., 2021) and news elaboration (Eveland, 2001) as predictors. Lee et al. (2020) found that COVID-19 misinformation exposure was positively associated with misbeliefs about COVID-19 but negatively associated with related knowledge; in their study, South Korean respondents who saw COVID-19 misinformation more often reported poorer knowledge about COVID-19. Among those who took less cognitive effort in elaborating on the information, misbeliefs were higher.

In addition to individual factors, the socio-political system of a society—and access to digital information in particular—can also affect how people access and learn from the media. In an environment where access to updated COVID-19 information is free and timely, citizens are more likely to filter out debunked misinformation as they find it easier to seek factually correct information, thus forming accurate perceptions as true beliefs from the message stimuli and gaining some knowledge about COVID-19. According to the analytical framework presented in Chapter 1, we expected that information accessibility as a macro factor would account for the differences in the cognitive outcomes from exposure to COVID-19 misinformation. That is, if misinformation can be deliberatively discussed or easily debunked, the negative cognitive effects could be attenuated.

Findings

Misbeliefs about COVID-19

To measure misbeliefs, we asked the 4,094 respondents to rate to what extent they believed the following five items are true: (1) COVID-19 virus can spread through 5G mobile networks; (2) Drinking bleach can kill COVID-19 virus; (3) Eating garlic can prevent COVID-19 infection; (4) COVID-19 vaccines will affect fertility; (5) COVID-19 vaccines will alter human DNA. The scale ranged from 1 to 5, where 1 = definitely false and 5 = definitely true. The five items were averaged to generate an index of misbeliefs about COVID-19

(M = 1.82, SD = 0.96). Thus, the higher score, the stronger misbeliefs about the COVID-19 pandemic.

Results of frequency analysis show that among the five misinformation items, "COVID-19 vaccines will affect fertility" (M = 2.01, SD = 1.15) and "COVID-19 vaccines will alter human DNA" (M = 1.97, SD = 1.16) were relatively high in being accepted as true. More than one-fifth (22.80%) of the 4,094 respondents formed misbeliefs about at least one of the five misinformation items.

Gender and Misbeliefs

To explore the possibility of a gender difference in misbeliefs about COVID-19, we conducted a series of independent t-tests on the averaged index. Females held more misbeliefs than males—on four of the five misinformation items, females showed higher beliefs. However, the gender differences in each item and the combined index were non-significant (t = 0.41, p > .05), indicating that misbeliefs about COVID-19 are of equal prevalence among males (M = 1.82, SD = 0.97) and females (M = 1.82, SD = 0.95).

Age and Misbeliefs

To explore whether the misbeliefs differed across age groups, we split the age scale at the median (39-year-old) to create two groups of younger (39-year-old or younger; n = 2,051) and older respondents (40-year-old or older; n = 2,042). As Table 8.1 shows, age differences existed—the overall misbelief score was higher among younger adults (M = 1.88, SD = 1.00) than older adults (M = 1.77, SD = 0.91), t = –3.63, p < .001. On four of five individual

Table 8.1 Differences in misbeliefs about COVID-19 between younger and older adults

	Younger adults (n = 2,051)	Older adults (n = 2,042)	t value
	M (SD)	M (SD)	
1 COVID-19 virus can spread through 5G mobile networks	1.69 (1.15)	1.59 (1.03)	–3.08**
2 Drinking bleach can kill COVID-19 virus	1.64 (1.17)	1.52 (1.05)	–3.38***
3 Eating garlic can prevent COVID-19 infection	1.91 (1.19)	1.90 (1.11)	–0.10
4 COVID-19 vaccines will affect fertility	2.11 (1.20)	1.92 (1.08)	–5.31***
5 COVID-19 vaccines will alter human DNA	2.03 (1.21)	1.91(1.12)	–3.53***
Combined index	1.88 (1.00)	1.77 (0.91)	–3.63***

Note: The items were rated from 1 to 5, where 1 = definitely false and 5 = definitely true; **p < .01, ***p < .001; t values are calculated based on the mean score differences; The age entry has one missing value.

misinformation items, younger adults proved significantly more vulnerable than older adults regarding misinformation. The fact that young people, who spend more time on social media than do older people, may explain why they were more likely to be influenced by the widely circulated misinformation online.

Education and Misbeliefs

To investigate whether misbeliefs about COVID-19 are associated with education level, we distinguished high and low-education respondents by splitting the education-level scale at the median (Bachelor's degree). More than one-third of the 4,094 respondents were classified into the low education group (n = 1,528; lower than bachelor's degree) and the remainder into the high education group (n = 2,566). Overall, misbelief differences were not significant by education level (low education: M = 1.83, SD = 0.91; high education: M = 1.81, SD = 0.99; t = −.66, p > .05). An exception was the item that "COVID-19 vaccines will alter human DNA"; the low-education group (M = 2.02, SD = 1.14) showed higher misbeliefs than did the high-education group (M = 1.94, SD = 1.18), t = −2.13, p < .05. This implies that people with high education level could be more suspicious to misinformation on vaccinations. Nevertheless, as Bronstein and Vinogradov (2021) argued, education alone is insufficient to combat online misinformation.

Exposure and Misbeliefs

To investigate whether exposure to COVID-19 misinformation was associated with level of misbeliefs, we distinguished high- and low-exposure respondents by splitting the exposure scale at the median (1.60). Nearly half of the 4,094 respondents were classified into the low-exposure group (n = 1,858; exposure score < 1.6) and the remainder into the high-exposure group (n = 2,236; refer to Chapter 4 for specific measures). In Table 8.2, the results of independent-sample t-tests show that misbeliefs were higher in the group with high misinformation-exposure frequency (M = 2.13, SD = 1.10) compared to the group with less frequent misinformation exposure (M = 1.45, SD = 0.97), t = 24.02, p < .001. The difference between high and low misinformation exposure level was consistent across all misinformation items. The results imply that misinformation exposure can be an important contributing factor in forming misbeliefs about COVID-19, which is consistent with previous literature that repetition is effective in persuasion (Allport & Lepkin, 1945).

Sharing and Misbeliefs

As discussed in Chapter 5, sharing digital information has become a major form of social media interaction. Sharing misinformation will lead to greater harms by confusing or misleading more people. In addition to affecting the receiver, sharing behavior could also exert effects on the information sender.

Table 8.2 Differences in misbeliefs about COVID-19 between individuals of low and high misinformation exposure

	Low exposure (n = 1,858)	High exposure (n = 2,235)	t value
	M (SD)	M (SD)	
1 COVID-19 virus can spread through 5G mobile networks	1.25 (0.70)	1.97 (1.24)	22.40***
2 Drinking bleach can kill COVID-19 virus	1.16 (0.56)	1.93 (1.32)	23.40***
3 Eating garlic can prevent COVID-19 infection	1.55 (0.88)	2.20 (1.26)	18.83***
4 COVID-19 vaccines will affect fertility	1.69 (0.92)	2.28 (1.24)	17.10***
5 COVID-19 vaccines will alter human DNA	1.62 (.91)	2.26 (1.27)	18.44***
Combined index	1.45 (0.57)	2.13 (1.10)	24.02***

Note: The items were rated from 1 to 5, where 1 = definitely false and 5 = definitely true; $**p < .01$, $***p < .001$; t values are calculated based on the mean score differences.

For example, sharing with the purpose of convincing others that the information may be true will be more likely to accumulate misbeliefs and make the information senders further ignore updated factual knowledge (Oyserman & Dawson, 2020). Thus, it seemed likely that frequency of sharing misinformation could reinforce people's false beliefs about the information.

To investigate whether sharing COVID-19 misinformation was associated with level of misbeliefs, we distinguished respondents with high- and low-sharing frequency by splitting sharing scale at the median (2.00). Nearly half of the 4,094 respondents were classified into the low-sharing group (n = 2,337; sharing frequency score $\leq$ 2.00) and the remainder into the high-sharing group (n = 1,757; refer to Chapter 5 for detailed measures). The results of independent-sample t-tests (Table 8.3) show that misbeliefs were higher in the group with high misinformation-sharing frequency (M = 2.14, SD = 1.12) compared to the group with less frequent misinformation exposure (M = 1.58, SD = 0.73), t = 19.50, $p < .001$. The difference between high and low misinformation-sharing levels was consistent across all five items.

Elaboration and Misbeliefs

According to Eveland (2001)'s cognitive elaboration model, elaboration, as the information processing of the news, can predict learning outcomes. Thus, we asked, could higher elaboration on misinformation make an audience more reflective about information, debunk misinformation, and lead to lower misbeliefs? We sought to answer this by distinguishing between respondents with high and low elaborative efforts, using the median (3.75) of the elaboration scale as the cutting-off point. The scale relied on four times as measures on a five-point Likert scale (1 = "strongly disagree" and 5 = "strongly agree"): After

Table 8.3 Differences in misbeliefs about COVID-19 between individuals of low and high misinformation sharing

	Low sharing (n = 2,337)	High sharing (n = 1,756)	t value
	M (SD)	M (SD)	
1 COVID-19 virus can spread through 5G mobile networks	1.34 (0.80)	2.05 (1.28)	21.88***
2 Drinking bleach can kill COVID-19 virus	1.30 (0.80)	1.96 (1.34)	19.54***
3 Eating garlic can prevent COVID-19 infection	1.67 (0.98)	2.21 (1.28)	15.28***
4 COVID-19 vaccines will affect fertility	1.83 (1.02)	2.25 (1.25)	11.95***
5 COVID-19 vaccines will alter human DNA	1.76 (1.02)	2.25 (1.28)	13.60***
Combined index	1.58 (.73)	2.14 (1.12)	19.50***

Note: The items were rated from 1 to 5, where 1 = definitely false and 5 = definitely true; $**p < .01$, $***p < .001$; t values are calculated based on the mean score differences.

exposure to misinformation about COVID-19, (1) I have thought about the issue of misinformation; (2) I have thought about its impact on the pandemic; (3) I have thought about consequences of misinformation; and (4) I often think about how COVID-19 misinformation relates to other COVID-19 information I know. The items were averaged to form a composite measure ($M = 3.71$, $SD = .76$, $\alpha = .86$). Nearly half of the 4,094 respondents were classified into the low-elaboration group ($n = 2,115$; elaboration score ≤ 3.75) and the remainder into the high-elaboration group ($n = 1,979$).

Table 8.4 shows the results of independent-sample t-tests found no significant differences in misbeliefs between the groups with low misinformation elaboration efforts ($M = 1.84$, $SD = 0.85$) and high misinformation-elaboration efforts ($M = 1.81$ $SD = 1.06$), $t = -1.11$, $p > .05$.

Although the results did not show significant effects of elaboration, they hinted at the necessity for future investigation. For example, on items like "COVID-19 vaccines will affect fertility" (low elaboration: $M = 2.06$, $SD = 1.08$; high elaboration: $M = 1.96$, $SD = 1.21$; $t = -3.04$, $p < .01$) and "COVID-19 vaccines will alter human DNA" (low elaboration: $M = 2.00$, $SD = 1.07$; high elaboration: $M = 1.94$, $SD = 1.26$; $t = -1.75$, $p > .05$), the high elaboration group showed a comparatively lower level of misbelief.

Cross-City Differences in Misbeliefs

As we discussed earlier, a social-political system, especially the digital media accessibility of a society, can affect how people access and learn from news, which in turn makes a difference in their misbeliefs. Thus, how did respondents from the four Asian cities differ in the misbeliefs level?

Table 8.4 Differences in misbeliefs about COVID-19 between individuals of low and high misinformation elaboration

	Low elaboration (n = 2,114)	High elaboration (n = 1,979)	t value
	M (SD)	M (SD)	
1 COVID-19 virus can spread through 5G mobile networks	1.63 (0.99)	1.65 (1.19)	0.61
2 Drinking bleach can kill COVID-19 virus	1.57 (1.01)	1.60 (1.22)	0.78
3 Eating garlic can prevent COVID-19 infection	1.93 (1.08)	1.88 (1.22)	–1.15
4 COVID-19 vaccines will affect fertility	2.06 (1.08)	1.96 (1.21)	–3.04**
5 COVID-19 vaccines will alter human DNA	2.00 (1.07)	1.94 (1.26)	–1.75
Combined index	1.84 (0.85)	1.81 (1.06)	–1.11

Note: The items were rated from 1 to 5, where 1 = definitely false and 5 = definitely true; **$p <$ .01, ***$p <$ .001; t values are calculated based on the mean score differences.

As shown in Table 8.5, the results of the ANOVA analysis indicated significant differences regarding COVID-19 misbeliefs among the four Asian cities, $F(3, 4090) = 70.94$, $p <$ .001. Specifically, Taipei respondents ($M = 1.69$, $SD = 0.89$) reported significantly lower misbeliefs compared with Hong Kong ($M = 1.85$, $SD = 0.87$), Beijing ($M = 1.85$, $SD = 1.06$), and Singapore ($M = 1.90$, $SD = 0.99$). As expected, respondents in Taipei, who enjoy the most democratic political system and freest access to digital media, had the least misbeliefs about the pandemic.

Predictors of Misbeliefs

Finally, we performed a hierarchical regression analysis to examine which of the independent variables—demographics, information accessibility, exposure to COVID-19 misinformation, misinformation sharing, misinformation elaboration—would have the most impact on misbeliefs.

As shown in Table 8.6, age was a significant but negative predictor of misbeliefs ($\beta = -.04$, $p <$ .05), indicating that older adults are not that easily convinced by COVID-19 misinformation compared to the younger adults. Access to digital information ($\beta = .02$, $p >$ .05) was not significantly associated with the misbeliefs. The result is consistent with the ANOVA results on cross-societal comparisons. Beijing, as the city with lowest information accessibility, did not differ much compared to Hong Kong and Singapore in terms of respondents' misbeliefs about COVID-19. Misinformation exposure ($\beta = .57$, $p <$ .001) and sharing ($\beta = .17$, $p <$ .001) were positive predictors of misbeliefs, while cognitive elaboration was a negative predictor ($\beta = -.11$, $p <$ .001). In fact, exposure was the strongest among all predictors, suggesting

Table 8.5 Differences in misbeliefs about COVID-19 among respondents from Beijing, Hong Kong, Taipei, and Singapore

	Beijing (n = 1,032)	Hong Kong (n = 1,017)	Taipei (n = 1,019)	Singapore (n = 1,025)	Total	F value
	M (SD)	M (SD)	M (SD)	M (SD)	M (SD)	
1 COVID-19 virus can spread through 5G mobile networks	1.74 (1.15)	1.66 (1.06)	1.46 (.97)	1.71 (1.16)	1.64 (1.09)	13.54***
2 Drinking bleach can kill COVID-19 virus	1.75 (1.24)	1.54 (1.05)	1.42 (.98)	1.62 (1.15)	1.58 (1.11)	15.26***
3 Eating garlic can prevent COVID-19 infection	1.97 (1.22)	1.82 (1.06)	1.91 (1.12)	1.93 (1.19)	1.91 (1.15)	3.10*
4 COVID-19 vaccines will affect fertility	1.91 (1.17)	2.15 (1.11)	1.83 (1.12)	2.16 (1.14)	2.01 (1.15)	21.77***
5 COVID-19 vaccines will alter human DNA	1.88 (1.20)	2.08 (1.10)	1.82 (1.13)	2.09 (1.19)	1.97 (1.16)	14.40***
Combined index	1.85 (1.06)	1.85 (0.87)	1.69 (0.89)	1.90 (0.99)	1.82 (0.96)	9.25***

Note: The items were rated from 1 to 5, where 1 = definitely false and 5 = definitely true; **$p < .01$, ***$p < .001$; t values are calculated based on the mean score differences.

the harm of misinformation exposure and active engagement in forming misbeliefs, while elaboration reduces it.

Knowledge about COVID-19

To measure knowledge about COVID-19, we asked the respondents to answer six multiple-choice questions (one out of four choices should be correct): (1) Who is the Director-General of WHO (World Health Organization) in fighting COVID pandemic (correct rate 66.10%)? (2) What is the approximate death rate of COVID-19 (Correct rate 39.50%)? (3) Which of the following figures is closest to the reported cases of COVID-19 globally by now (correct rate 53.20%)? (4) To have the best vaccination effect, what is the recommended time for us to take the second dose following the first shot of COVID-19 vaccine (correct rate 62.30%)? (5) To ensure equitable access to COVID-19 vaccine, WHO has initiated a global scheme to allow rich countries to share COVID-19 vaccines with poor countries. What is the name

Table 8.6 Hierarchical regression analysis predicting misbeliefs about COVID-19

Predictors	Misbeliefs
Block 1: Demographics	
Age	.03*
Gender (Male = 1)	−.03*
Education	−.03*
City (Beijing = 1)	−.14***
Adjusted R²	0.0%
Block 2: Misinformation exposure	
Misinformation exposure	.53***
Incremental adjusted R²	30.0%
Block 3: Misinformation sharing	
Misinformation sharing	.19***
Incremental adjusted R²	2.6%
Block 4: Elaboration	
Elaboration	−.11***
Incremental adjusted R²	1.0%
Total adjusted R²	33.6%

Note: N = 4,093; *p < .05, ***p < .001; Beijing is coded as 1 and other cities are coded as 0; The age entry has one missing value.

of the scheme (correct rate 53.50%)? (6) According to the naming schemes of WHO, which one of the following items is not the variant of COVID-19 virus that has been found and identified by WHO (correct rate 51.30%)?

One point was added if the respondent correctly answered one question. The total score on six items was summed up to measure knowledge level. Overall, the mean score of the respondents' knowledge level was 2.64 (*median* = 1.82, *mode* = 3.00, *SD* = 1.53, *range* = 0.00–5.00). Among the 4,094 respondents, 9.60% scored zero points while 13.20% reported 5 points. No one was able to answer all questions correctly.

Gender and Knowledge

To explore whether knowledge on COVID-19 differed between gender, an independent *t*-test was conducted on the summed knowledge scores. As shown in Table 8.7, the gender difference was significant ($t = -10.10$, $p < .001$). In general, males ($M = 2.88$, $SD = 1.57$) had a higher knowledge score than females ($M = 2.41$, $SD = 1.46$).

In addition, we conducted a series of chi-square tests to explore the gender differences on correct rates of each item. Results showed that on each question, a higher percentage of males answered correctly than did the females. For instance, on the question "Who is the Director-General of WHO (World Health Organization) in fighting COVID pandemic," 71.5% of males answered correctly while only 61.1% of females answered correctly, χ2 (1, N = 4094) = 49.68, $p < .001$.

Table 8.7 Gender differences in knowledge about COVID-19

	Males Correct (%)	Females Correct (%)	χ^2
1 Who is the Director-General of WHO (World Health Organization) in fighting COVID pandemic?	71.5%	61.1%	49.68***
2 What is the approximate death rate of COVID-19?	45.5%	33.9%	57.24***
3 Which of the following figures is closest to the reported cases of COVID-19 globally by now?	58.2%	48.6%	37.91***
4 To have the best vaccination effect, what is the recommended time for us to take the second dose following the first shot of COVID-19 vaccine?	64.1%	60.6%	5.25*
5 To ensure equitable access to COVID-19 vaccine, WHO has initiated a global scheme to allow rich countries to share COVID-19 vaccines with poor countries. What is the name of the scheme?	57.7%	49.7%	26.41***
6 According to the naming schemes of WHO, which one of the following items is not the variant of COVID-19 virus that has been founded and identified by WHO?	55.6%	51.3%	27.89***
	M (SD)	*M (SD)*	*t value*
Combined index of knowledge	2.88(1.57)	2.41(1.46)	−10.10***

Note: $*p < .05$, $***p < .001$.

Age and Knowledge

To explore age differences in knowledge about COVID-19, we split the age scale at the median (39-year-old) to create two groups of younger ($n = 2,051$; 18–39 years old) and older respondents ($n = 2,042$; 40–85 years old). Table 8.8 shows that the average knowledge score was higher among older adults ($M = 2.78$, $SD = 1.55$) than younger adults ($M = 2.50$, $SD = 1.51$), $t = 5.84$, $p < .001$.

Concerning the correct rates, older adults performed better than youngsters on the other four questions. For instance, on the question about the approximate death rate of COVID-19 at the fieldwork time, 44% of the older adults submitted the right answer while 35.0% of the younger adults answered correctly, $\chi2$ $(1, N = 4093) = 34.58$, $p < .001$.

Education and Knowledge

To investigate whether knowledge was associated with education level, we distinguished high- and low-education respondents by splitting the education-level scale at the median (bachelor's degree). More than 1/3 of the

Table 8.8 Differences in knowledge about COVID-19 between younger and older adults

	Younger adults Correct (%)	Older adults Correct (%)	χ^2
1 Who is the Director-General of WHO (World Health Organization) in fighting COVID pandemic?	60.5%	71.8%	59.02***
2 What is the approximate death rate of COVID-19?	35.0%	44.0%	34.58***
3 Which of the following figures is closest to the reported cases of COVID-19 globally by now?	53.6%	52.8%	.24
4 To have the best vaccination effect, what is the recommended time for us to take the second dose following the first shot of COVID-19 vaccine?	63.2%	61.4%	1.41
5 To ensure equitable access to COVID-19 vaccine, WHO has initiated a global scheme to allow rich countries to share COVID-19 vaccines with poor countries. What is the name of the scheme?	51.9%	55.2%	4.46*
6 According to the naming schemes of WHO, which one of the following items is not the variant of COVID-19 virus that has been founded and identified by WHO?	48.8%	53.8%	10.40***
	M (SD)	*M (SD)*	*t* value
Combined index of knowledge	2.50(1.51)	2.78(1.55)	5.84***

Note: $*p < .05$, $***p < .001$.

4,094 respondents were classified into the low-education group ($n = 1,528$; lower than bachelor's degree) and the remainder into the high-education group ($n = 2,566$). As Table 8.9 shows, overall, there was a significant difference between the low- and high-education groups on their knowledge score (low education: $M = 2.23$, $SD = 1.54$; high education: $M = 2.88$, $SD = 1.48$; $t = 13.27$, $p < .001$). In addition, on each individual question, the high-education group scored a higher correct rate than did the low-education group. For instance, on the question about the COVID-19 variant, 57% of the high-education group answered correctly while only 41.70% of the low-education group answered correctly, χ^2 (1, N = 4094) = 90.05, $p < .001$.

The results show some differences compared with the relationship between education and misinformation belief. Although the mean score of misbeliefs did not differ between high- and low-education levels, the mean score of knowledge showed a significant difference. In other words, education may not be a powerful weapon in combating widely spread misinformation on social media but is still useful in helping people know more about the issue and news topics.

Table 8.9 Differences in knowledge about COVID-19 between individuals of low and high education

	Low education Correct (%)	High education Correct (%)	χ^2
1 Who is the Director-General of WHO (World Health Organization) in fighting COVID pandemic?	58.3%	70.8%	66.82***
2 What is the approximate death rate of COVID-19?	33.1%	43.3%	41.86***
3 Which of the following figures is closest to the reported cases of COVID-19 globally by now?	45.8%	57.6%	53.81***
4 To have the best vaccination effect, what is the recommended time for us to take the second dose following the first shot of COVID-19 vaccine?	65.5%	60.4%	10.63***
5 To ensure equitable access to COVID-19 vaccine, WHO has initiated a global scheme to allow rich countries to share COVID-19 vaccines with poor countries. What is the name of the scheme?	44.4%	59.0%	81.24***
6 According to the naming schemes of WHO, which one of the following items is not the variant of COVID-19 virus that has been founded and identified by WHO?	41.7%	57.0%	90.05***
	M (SD)	M (SD)	*t* value
Combined index of knowledge	2.23(1.54)	2.88(1.48)	13.27***

Note: ***$p < .001$.

Exposure to Misinformation and Knowledge

To investigate whether exposure to COVID-19 misinformation was associated with level of COVID-19 knowledge, we distinguished high- and low-exposure respondents by splitting the exposure scale at the median (1.60). Nearly half of the 4,094 respondents were classified into the low-exposure group ($n = 1,858$; exposure score < 1.6) and the remainder into the high-exposure group ($n = 2,236$). As noted in Table 8.10, the results of independent-sample *t*-tests showed that the group with low misinformation exposure frequency had a higher knowledge level ($M = 2.70$, $SD = 1.51$) compared to the group with more frequent misinformation exposure ($M = 2.58$, $SD = 1.55$). The difference was significant ($t = -2.56$, $p < .05$).

In addition, concerning the correct answer rate, no differences existed between the high- and low-exposure groups on half of the items. On two out of the six questions, the low-exposure group had a higher correct rate than

Table 8.10 Differences in knowledge about COVID-19 between individuals of low and high misinformation exposure

	Low exposure Correct (%)	High exposure Correct (%)	χ^2
1 Who is the Director-General of WHO (World Health Organization) in fighting COVID pandemic?	70.1%	62.9%	23.46***
2 What is the approximate death rate of COVID-19?	39.7%	39.4%	.03
3 Which of the following figures is closest to the reported cases of COVID-19 globally by now?	50.5%	55.5%	9.86**
4 To have the best vaccination effect, what is the recommended time for us to take the second dose following the first shot of COVID-19 vaccine?	62.3%	62.3%	.00
5 To ensure equitable access to COVID-19 vaccine, WHO has initiated a global scheme to allow rich countries to share COVID-19 vaccines with poor countries. What is the name of the scheme?	54.0%	53.1%	.34
6 According to the naming schemes of WHO, which one of the following items is not the variant of COVID-19 virus that has been founded and identified by WHO?	56.1%	47.3%	31.91***
	M (SD)	*M (SD)*	*t value*
Combined index of knowledge	2.70(1.51)	2.58(1.55)	−2.56*

Note: *p < .05, **p < .01, ***p < .001.

did the high-exposure group. For instance, on the COVID-19 variant question, only 47.3% of the high-exposure group answered correctly while only 56.1% of the low-exposure group answered correctly, χ^2 (1, N = 4094) = 31.91, p < .001).

Misinformation Sharing and Knowledge

As discussed, not only exposure to but also sharing misinformation may lead to higher misbeliefs. Then what would be the effects of misinformation sharing on knowledge? Again, we distinguished respondents with high- and low-sharing frequency by splitting sharing scale at the median (2.00). Nearly half of the 4,094 respondents were classified into the low-sharing group (n = 2,337; sharing frequency score ≤ 2.00) and the remainder into the high-sharing group (n = 1,757). The results of independent-sample t-tests (see Table 8.11) show that the group with high misinformation-sharing frequency recorded a lower knowledge score (M = 2.34, SD = 1.53) compared to the group with less frequent misinformation sharing ($M = 2.86$, $SD = 1.50$). The difference was significant ($t = -10.98$, $p < .001$).

Further, on each question, the correct percentage was higher in the low-sharing group compared with the high-sharing group. For example, on the question about COVID-19 vaccine scheme, 55.5% of the low-sharing group answered correctly while 51.0% of the high-sharing group got the right answer, $\chi2$ (1, N= 4094) = 8.02, $p < .01$.

Elaboration and Knowledge

To investigate whether higher elaboration could lead to higher knowledge level, we distinguished respondents by high and low elaborative efforts. Elaboration scale was split at the median (3.75). Nearly half of the 4,094 respondents were classified into the low-elaboration group ($n = 2,115$; elaboration score ≤ 3.75) and the remainder into the high-elaboration group ($n = 1,979$).

Table 8.11 Differences in knowledge about COVID-19 between individuals of low and high misinformation sharing

	Low sharing Correct (%)	High sharing Correct (%)	χ^2
1 Who is the Director-General of WHO (World Health Organization) in fighting COVID pandemic?	73.0%	57.0%	115.67***
2 What is the approximate death rate of COVID-19?	43.3%	34.4%	33.33***
3 Which of the following figures is closest to the reported cases of COVID-19 globally by now?	54.8%	51.2%	5.23*
4 To have the best vaccination effect, what is the recommended time for us to take the second dose following the first shot of COVID-19 vaccine?	60.3%	64.9%	9.06**
5 To ensure equitable access to COVID-19 vaccine, WHO has initiated a global scheme to allow rich countries to share COVID-19 vaccines with poor countries. What is the name of the scheme?	55.5%	51.0%	8.02**
6 According to the naming schemes of WHO, which one of the following items is not the variant of COVID-19 virus that has been founded and identified by WHO?	59.6%	40.2%	150.58***
	M (SD)	*M (SD)*	*t* value
Combined index of knowledge	2.86(1.50)	2.34(1.53)	-10.98***

Note: *p < .05, **p < .01, ***p < .001.

As the results of independent-samples *t*-tests in Table 8.12 show, the average knowledge score for the group with low misinformation elaboration efforts (*M* = 2.45, *SD* = 1.54was significantly lower than that of the group with high-misinformation elaboration efforts (*M* = 2.83, *SD* = 1.51). The difference was significant (*t* = 7.87, *p* < .001). Further, the high-elaboration group recorded a significantly higher proportion of correct answers for five of the six questions. For instance, on the question about the COVID-19 death rate, 42.4% of the high-elaboration group answered correctly; while only 36.8% of the low-elaboration group answered correctly, $\chi2$ (1, *N* = 4094) = 13.38, *p* < .001.

Table 8.12 Differences in knowledge about COVID-19 between individuals of low and high misinformation elaboration

	Low elaboration Correct (%)	*High elaboration* Correct (%)	χ^2
1 Who is the Director-General of WHO (World Health Organization) in fighting COVID pandemic?	64.0%	68.4%	8.51**
2 What is the approximate death rate of COVID-19?	36.8%	42.4%	13.38***
3 Which of the following figures is closest to the reported cases of COVID-19 globally by now?	49.6%	57.1%	22.96***
4 To have the best vaccination effect, what is the recommended time for us to take the second dose following the first shot of COVID-19 vaccine?	61.9%	62.7%	0.27
5 To ensure equitable access to COVID-19 vaccine, WHO has initiated a global scheme to allow rich countries to share COVID-19 vaccines with poor countries. What is the name of the scheme?	46.6%	60.9%	84.56***
6 According to the naming schemes of WHO, which one of the following items is not the variant of COVID-19 virus that has been founded and identified by WHO?	48.5%	54.3%	13.46***
	M (SD)	*M (SD)*	*t value*
Combined index of knowledge	2.45(1.54)	2.83(1.51)	7.87***

Note: **p < .01, ***p < .001.

Misbeliefs and Knowledge

To investigate whether COVID-19 misbelief was associated with the level of COVID-19 knowledge, we distinguished high- and low-misinformation belief by splitting the misbelief scale at the median (1.40). Nearly half of the 4,094 respondents were classified into the low-misbelief group (n = 2,066; misbelief score ≤ 1.40) and the remainder into the high-misbelief group (n = 2,028). As Table 8.13 shows, the results of independent-sample t-tests of knowledge were significant (t = 14.15, p < .001) between the group with high misbeliefs and low misbeliefs. The high group's knowledge level was lower (M = 2.30, SD = 1.53) than the group with low misbeliefs (M = 2.97, SD = 1.47). Further, for five of the six questions, the low-misbelief group recorded a significantly higher proportion of correct answers. For example, on the question about the WHO Director-General, 73.20% of the low-misbelief group answered correctly while only 58.90% of the high-misbelief group answered correctly, $\chi2$ (1, N = 4094) = 93.36, p < .001.

Table 8.13 Differences in knowledge about COVID-19 between individuals of low and high misbeliefs

	Low misbeliefs Correct (%)	High misbeliefs Correct (%)	χ^2
1 Who is the Director-General of WHO (World Health Organization) in fighting COVID pandemic?	73.2%	58.9%	93.36***
2 What is the approximate death rate of COVID-19?	45.8%	33.1%	69.32***
3 Which of the following figures is closest to the reported cases of COVID-19 globally by now?	57.7%	48.7%	33.70***
4 To have the best vaccination effect, what is the recommended time for us to take the second dose following the first shot of COVID-19 vaccine?	63.3%	61.2%	1.92
5 To ensure equitable access to COVID-19 vaccine, WHO has initiated a global scheme to allow rich countries to share COVID-19 vaccines with poor countries. What is the name of the scheme?	59.9%	47.1%	67.01***
6 According to the naming schemes of WHO, which one of the following items is not the variant of COVID-19 virus that has been founded and identified by WHO?	60.0%	42.5%	124.66***
	M (SD)	M (SD)	t value
Combined index of knowledge	2.97(1.47)	2.30(1.53)	14.15***

Note: **p < .01, ***p < .001.

Cross-City Differences in COVID-19 Knowledge

To explore differences on knowledge levels among respondents from the four cities, we conducted ANOVA analyses. Results are presented in Table 8.14. They show significant differences among the four cities, $F(3, 4090) = 105.88$, $p < .001$. Specifically, Taipei respondents ($M = 3.28$, $SD = 1.43$) had a significantly higher knowledge score, followed by Hong Kong ($M = 2.71$, $SD = 1.45$), Singapore ($M = 2.31$, $SD = 1.57$), and Beijing ($M = 2.25$, $SD = 1.46$).

Except for the question on vaccination timing, Taipei respondents scored a higher correct percentage. For example, on the question about number of reported COVID-19 cases globally, 65.9% respondents from Taipei answered correctly, while 57.1% Beijing respondents, 52.8% Hong Kong respondents, and 37.2% Singapore respondents got the right answer, $\chi2$ (3, $N = 4094$) = 178.58, $p < .001$.

Table 8.14 Differences in knowledge about COVID-19 among respondents from Beijing, Hong Kong, Taipei, and Singapore

	Beijing (n = 1,032)	Hong Kong (n = 1,017)	Taipei (n = 1,019)	Singapore (n = 1,025)	Total	χ^2
	Correct (%)	Correct (%)	Correct (%)	Correct (%)	Correct (%)	
1 Who is the Director-General of WHO (World Health Organization) in fighting COVID pandemic?	48.1%	75.9%	83.7%	57.2%	66.1%	371.2***
2 What is the approximate death rate of COVID-19?	38.4%	41.4%	43.6%	34.7%	39.5%	18.90***
3 Which of the following figures is closest to the reported cases of COVID-19 globally by now?	57.1%	52.8%	65.9%	37.2%	53.2%	178.58***
4 To have the best vaccination effect, what is the recommended time for us to take the second dose following the first shot of COVID-19 vaccine?	76.3%	75.5%	27.7%	69.6%	62.3%	704.45***

(Continued)

Table 8.14 Continued

	Beijing (n = 1,032)	Hong Kong (n = 1,017)	Taipei (n = 1,019)	Singapore (n = 1,025)	Total	χ^2
	Correct (%)	Correct (%)	Correct (%)	Correct (%)	Correct (%)	
5 Which of the following figures is closest to the reported cases of COVID-19 globally by now?	45.5%	47.9%	69.6%	51.2%	53.5%	147.19***
6 According to the naming schemes of WHO, which one of the following items is not the variant of COVID-19 virus that has been founded and identified by WHO?	35.9%	53.5%	65.4%	50.6%	51.3%	180.08***
	M (SD)	M (SD)	M (SD)	M (SD)	M (SD)	F value
Combined index of knowledge	2.25(1.46)	2.71(1.45)	3.28(1.43)	2.31(1.57)	2.64(1.53)	105.88***

Note: ***$p < .001$; F values are calculated based on one way ANOVA test on the mean score difference.

Predictors of COVID-19 Knowledge

Finally, we performed a hierarchical regression analysis to examine which of the independent variables—demographics, information accessibility, exposure to and sharing of misinformation, misinformation elaboration, and misbeliefs—would have the most impact on knowledge about COVID-19. As the results in Table 8.15 show, all major demographic factors were significant predictors of COVID-19 knowledge, including age ($\beta = .14$, $p < .001$), gender ($\beta = .13$, $p < .001$), and education ($\beta = .24$, $p < .001$). Older males with higher education proved better at COVID-19 knowledge. Also, information accessibility ($\beta = -.15$, $p < .001$) was significantly and positively associated with COVID-19 knowledge. Low information accessibility seemed to hinder Beijing respondents' ability to acquire knowledge about COVID-19.

Both misinformation exposure ($\beta = -.09$, $p < .001$) and sharing ($\beta = -.14$, $p < .001$) were negative predictors of knowledge, while cognitive elaboration was a positive predictor ($\beta = .15$, $p < .001$), suggesting that the passive exposure and active engagement were the barriers to knowledge gain, whereas cognitive elaboration was instrumental in gaining knowledge about the pandemic. In addition, misbeliefs were also a negative predictor of people's

Table 8.15 Hierarchical regression analysis predicting knowledge about COVID-19

Predictors	Knowledge
Block 1: Demographics	
Age	.13***
Gender (Male = 1)	.12***
Education	.21***
City (Beijing = 1)	−.16***
Adjusted R^2	10.7%
Block 2: Misinformation exposure	
Misinformation exposure	.09***
Incremental adjusted R^2	0.8%
Block 3: Misinformation sharing	
Misinformation sharing	−.10***
Incremental adjusted R^2	1.5%
Block 4: Elaboration	
Elaboration	.12***
Incremental adjusted R^2	2.1%
Block 5: Misbeliefs	
Misbeliefs	−.30***
Incremental adjusted R^2	6.1%
Total adjusted R^2	21.2%

Note: $N = 4,093$; ***$p < .001$; Beijing is coded as 1 and other cities are coded as 0; The age entry has one missing value.

knowledge ($\beta = -.30$, $p < .001$). Knowledge level could be the accumulated outcome of individual differences and misinformation experiences.

Summary of Key Findings

This chapter examined the adverse cognitive effects of misinformation on the dimension of false beliefs and knowledge about COVID-19. Our large-scale cross-societal analysis of misinformation in Beijing, Hong Kong, Taipei, and Singapore shows that viewing and sharing misinformation has resulted in harms on citizens' beliefs and knowledge in terms of altering perceptions and hindering the gain of knowledge about the pandemic. Specifically,

- Overall, although the misbelief score among the 4,094 respondents was not high, it was higher among certain demographic groups than others: misbeliefs are of equal level between males and females.
- Older respondents are less likely to form misbeliefs than are younger ones. They also have better knowledge of COVID-19 than the younger adults. Although the mean score of misbeliefs did not differ between high- and low-education levels, the mean score of knowledge showed a significant difference.

- High-misinformation exposure respondents have a higher misbelief score, but lower knowledge level compared with low-exposure respondents. Similarly, misinformation sharing, as the active engagement behavior, is positively related to people's misbeliefs and is negatively related to their knowledge level.
- Cognitive elaboration provides greatly increases the ability to reject misinformation—the more people elaborate on the misinformation, the less likely they will form misbeliefs and the more knowledgeable they will be about COVID-19.
- Compared to those with a lower level of misbeliefs, respondents with a higher level of misbeliefs also reported a lower level of COVID-19 knowledge.
- Respondents in Taipei, who enjoy the freest access to digital information and the marketplace of ideas, were less likely to form misbeliefs compared with those in Beijing, Hong Kong, and Singapore. As a result, Taipei respondents also had the highest average score of COVID-19 knowledge.
- When all factors are considered together, those that account for the differences in COVID-19 misbeliefs are age, misinformation exposure, sharing, and elaboration. In particular, misinformation exposure and sharing are the positive predictors of forming misbeliefs whereas elaboration is a negative predictor.
- Factors that account for the differences in COVID-19 knowledge are key demographics (i.e., age, gender, education), information accessibility, misinformation exposure, sharing, elaboration, and false beliefs. In particular, misinformation exposure, sharing, and misbeliefs are the negative predictors of acquiring knowledge whereas elaboration is a positive predictor.

Qualitative Findings

What to Believe?

It is said that knowledge knows no boundaries. However, politics, ideology, ignorance, and uncertainties may circumscribe knowledge. As reported in the quantitative findings section, the more that respondents read, including misinformation, the more misbeliefs they acquired. Insights from the thoughts and accounts of the participants shed light on how they screened information to filter out misinformation, that is, distinguishing falsehood from truth, and then making knowledge-based decisions when dealing with COVID.

In general, participants from Beijing, especially those aged 40 years or older, relied heavily on government announcements as the main source of COVID-19-related information. Many of them mentioned that no matter whether news came from Internet channels or from state-run TV, if it came from the government, they would consider it believable. Ms. Gao, a 44-year-old mother of two who also has a full-time job in education, shared with the group that she trusted the WeChat Account owned and managed by the

China's State Council the most. As she explained, "The news from there [the State Council] must be the most up-to-date, and the people who announce the news must be the most authoritative." Other Beijing participants also mentioned a few different government-managed apps, such as "Beijing Tong" (北京通), an 'Internet+ government service' system that pools data of 53 municipal agencies for timely and orderly sharing in the capital city.

Many participants from Singapore mentioned that the media were controlled by the government. Unlike Beijing participants' unanimous agreement on trusting such media, the Singaporeans' views were quite split. Half of them believed state media, half did not. Some of the Singaporeans in the group simply termed the news from non-government sources as "hoax." For example, Ella, a young female white-collar worker in fintech, cited a growing tide of influx of news.

> Sometimes I will point it out you know that it's fake, where did you get this from? Can you justify it? And the moment you cannot justify it coming from either government-owned platforms or our state news publishers, media platforms, and then, yeah, that's a hoax, basically.

However, Mason, a middle-aged father working in electronics, showed his concerns about how important information related to COVID vaccine might be covered up by the media. He explained,

> So actually there was quite a bit of concern after recent months of reports about the mRNA thing. I think there was some news or something about Pfizer. The key thing is I think that there are some reports and some stuff that information is not readily available locally because our media is quite restricted… some information that came from abroad… mentioned that the mRNA actually changes your DNA structure eventually. So yeah, that's one of the major concerns I have.

Unlike the media systems developed in Beijing and Singapore, where "government" in the news is often used as an abstract "totality term," the meaning of the "government" seems to be more concrete in Hong Kong. The focus group discussants usually referred to specific government entities or agencies such as "The Department of Health" or "The Fire Service Department" when they talked about the information sources that they trusted.

In addition, a number of senior participants also mentioned that they relied on and trusted the traditional news media more than online channels. Sofia, a 50-year-old female sales manager from Singapore, told the focus group that she still watched TV news from the mainstream media. Why? She said,

> I still have channel news, Asia (Channel NewsAsia, CAN), CNN News or Bloomberg News, which are more trustworthy, but not 100%. As I mentioned previously, they may not have all the updated data, but I

think they are good enough, trustworthy news that we can take it with a pinch of salt, some allowance for mistakes, but generally I think it's all right. This news is quite trustworthy.

In a similar way, Benjamin, a 58-year-old Hong Kong male accounting manager in Hong Kong, said the following about what to believe when it comes down to filtering a mass amount of information about COVID-19:

The information from the Department of Health is reliable. I wouldn't say so for other information sources because some of them are just passing false messages. Even on YouTube, you can find a lot of information about this pandemic, and the question remains whether you should believe it or not.

The participants' trust of the traditional media seemed to spill over to their own beliefs in and judgment about the safety of COVID-19 vaccines. As Mr. Xu, a 55-year-old male salesman in Beijing, explained,

A friend of mine told me that he thought the vaccine we [China] developed was unsafe... The safety of vaccine, as I just mentioned, has also been proven. That is to say, it went through the first phase of clinical trials and the second phase of clinical trials. These are some experiments conducted by the state, and they have been approved... It has been accounted and explained on TV and news for more than a year. There is no evidence to show that it is not safe.

It is also worth noting that the older generation in the focus groups tended to project everything (news, videos, etc.) from the "small screen" (e.g., the smartphone) onto the "big screen" (e.g., TV), and the distinction between the two, or "new vs. old" media, was actually quite blurred. As a consequence, even when the news was from the mobile media, if it was received (projected) on TV, the participants still thought it was believable.

Knowledge as Belief

Another insight from the focus group discussion is that knowledge itself is often loaded with values and beliefs of people who hold them. While individual participants might have been exposed to different information sources, or sharing information to different extents, once the information seemed to contradict their own beliefs, they started to challenge its authenticity. Ms. Chen, a 26-year-old female white collar from an upper-middle-class family in Beijing, shared her thoughts on such tendencies. She said, "For example, it was also posted on the Internet or WeChat moments before, when the outbreak in Shanghai was very serious, I often saw the news in the 'Circle of Friends' [on WeChat] that many people wrote stories about the pandemic in Shanghai. There are things that could be true. But I feel that some people may be deliberately creating panic, and they are talking about boards put up around the quarantine hotel being blown away by the wind, and so on. This is very negative, and it will damage the image of the country. I think, whether it is true or false, [it is] not easy to distinguish."

When there was a lack of sources to verify or to debunk the misinformation on social media, the participants indicated that they had to apply their "folk knowledge" to minimize the potential harm caused by misinformation even if such "folk knowledge" might not be reliable. Mr. Su, a 50-year-old male business owner from Taipei who rarely shared information online, mostly trusted the information sent by his younger brother. But whenever he received something from his father, he would use his own reasoning to differentiate what to trust and what to ignore. "Whatever my father passed on to me," he explained,

> like which food should be eaten with what, and which food could prevent COVID, I would say, food therapy, normal food, you can try; but if you have to buy some kind of traditional Chinese medicine, or if it's a quack remedy, absolutely not. He asked about something like garlic with lemon and honey, and I told him that these are natural things that you can try. But you should never buy something that I don't know what it is made of.

Insights and Implications for Public Policy

Previous research (e.g., Cho et al., 2009; Eveland, 2001) suggests the positive role of media for citizens to learn about politics and social issues. However, in the context of the global pandemic, widely circulated misinformation about COVID-19 on social media platforms seems to impede the public's acquisition of factual knowledge. The findings in this chapter have implications for containing the harmful effects of misinformation on citizens' cognitive capacities in dealing with misinformation surrounding COVID-19.

First, mobilizing the public to make cognitive efforts in processing debunked yet popular misinformation about COVID-19 seems to hold the key in reducing the impact of encountering misinformation on forming misbeliefs that negatively affect the level of people's knowledge about the new disease. Education could be a powerful tool in preparing and equipping the public to form accurate perceptions about the new disease.

In practice, the authorities and government public health agencies should acknowledge that knowledge is power in pandemic control and help the public to acquire knowledge about the pandemic through public education campaigns. In planning a campaign to stop the spread of misinformation and reduce its harms on the public, authorities should develop messages that facilitate the public's deep thinking or elaborative processing. While accurate knowledge can help build citizens' necessary literacy to cope with the disease, only when misbeliefs are reduced will fact-based knowledge increase.

In addition, the harmful effects of misinformation on COVID-19 on citizens' cognitive abilities in society appear to be differential, subject to the larger societal context—digital information accessibility. The negative cognitive effects of misinformation are less in societies with free access because citizens can access a diverse range of information to stay informed. However, in information-poor societies with restricted access, citizens cannot get rich information resources and tend to be harmed more by misinformation. Thus, our findings highlighted the importance of free flow of digital information.

Accordingly, public health authorities and medical experts should maintain open and transparent communication with the public, especially on digital media platforms. As soon as misinformation about COVID-19 appears on social media platforms, factual and evidence-based information should be presented quickly so that the general public can fact-check user-generated content to sort out inaccurate or false information. Timely and accurate information published from authorities' sources, such as health agencies, should reduce the chance of misinformation that affects the public's beliefs and knowledge.

References

Allport, F. H., & Lepkin, M. (1945). Wartime rumors of waste and special privilege: Why some people believe them. *The Journal of Abnormal and Social Psychology, 40*(1), 3–36.

Bronstein, M. V., & Vinogradov, S. (2021). Education alone is insufficient to combat online medical misinformation. *EMBO Reports, 22*(3), e52282. https://doi.org/10.15252/embr.202052282

Cho, J., Shah, D. V., McLeod, J. M., McLeod, D. M., Scholl, R. M., & Gotlieb, M. R. (2009).Campaigns, reflection, and deliberation: Advancing an OSROR model of communication effects. *Communication Theory, 19*(1), 66–88. https://doi.org/10.1111/j.1468-2885.2008.01333.x

Chong, S. K., Ali, S. H., Đoàn, L. N., Yi, S. S., Trinh-Shevrin, C., & Kwon, S. C. (2021). Social media use and misinformation among Asian Americans during COVID-19. *Frontiers in Public Health, 9.* https://www.ncbi.nlm.nih.gov/pmc/articles/PMC8795661/

Chou, W., Gaysynsky, A., & Cappellar, J. (2020). Where to go from here: Health misinformation on social media. *American Journal of Public Health, 110*(3), S273–S275. https://doi.org/10.2105/AJPH.2020.305905

Eveland, W. P. (2001). The cognitive mediation model of learning from the news: Evidence from nonelection, off-year election, and presidential election contexts. *Communication Research, 28*(5), 571–601. https://doi.org/10.1177/009365001028005001

Gerosa, T., Gui, M., Hargittai, E., & Nguyen, M. H. (2021). (Mis) informed during COVID-19: How education level and information sources contribute to knowledge gaps. *International Journal of Communication, 15*, 2196–2217. https://ijoc.org/index.php/ijoc/article/view/16438

Lee, J. J., Kang, K. A., Wang, M. P., Zhao, S. Z., Wong, J. Y. H., O'Connor, S., Yang, C. S., & Shin, S. (2020). Associations between COVID-19 misinformation exposure and belief with COVID-19 knowledge and preventive behaviors: Cross-sectional online study. *Journal of Medical Internet Research, 22*(11), e22205. http://dx.doi.org/10.2196/22205

McKinley, C. J., & Lauby, F. (2021). Anti-vaccine beliefs and COVID-19 information seeking on social media: Examining processes influencing COVID-19 beliefs and preventative actions. *International Journal of Communication, 15*, 4252–4274. https://ijoc.org/index.php/ijoc/article/view/17714

Oyserman, D., & Dawson, A. (2020). Your fake news, our facts: Identity-based motivation shapes what we believe, share, and accept. In *The psychology of fake news* (pp. 173–195). London: Routledge.

Pennycook, G., McPhetres, J., Zhang, Y., Lu, J. G., & Rand, D. G. (2020). Fighting COVID-19 misinformation on social media: Experimental evidence for a scalable accuracy-nudge intervention. *Psychological Science, 31*(7), 770–780. https://doi.org/10.1177/0956797620939054

Pluviano, S., Watt, C., & Della Sala, S. (2017). Misinformation lingers in memory: Failure of three pro-vaccination strategies. *PloS One, 12*(7), e0181640. https://doi.org/10.1371/journal.pone.0181640

Wei, R., Guo, J., Wang, S., & Yi-Hui, H. (2022). The role of digital information accessibility in shaping the relationships of exposure to COVID-19 misinformation and cognitive and attitudinal effects in Asia. *Communication and Society, 62*, 207–264. http://www.cschinese.com/issueArticle.asp?P_No=93&CA_ID=708

9 Swamped

Misinformation and Information Overload

Ran Wei, Wenting Yu, and Jing Guo

Introduction

Relying on Internet technology and digital information to cope with the disruptions in daily lives, work, and leisure caused by the lockdowns and quarantines since January 2020 has become a worldwide trend. As the global health crisis entered the third year, the level of public uncertainty, anxiety, and fatigue increased in Beijing, Hong Kong, Singapore, and Taipei. The cities implemented varying levels of strict pandemic control policies (ranging from Beijing's zero-tolerance approach to Singapore's living with COVID policy). Unprecedented time online and incessant COVID-19 information from endless cycles of updates on new variants on a daily basis have resulted in a state of COVID-19 information overload.

At the same time, there has been a general increase in active information avoidance, especially since the COVID-19 outbreaks. According to Reuters Institute data back in 2017, 29% of news users worldwide said they avoided news (Newman et al., 2017). In 2022, 38% of respondents reported they sometimes or often selectively avoided news (Newman et al., 2022). The most common reason for avoidance is "there is too much politics and COVID-19," implying that information overload could be a driving factor of information avoidance during the long-haul pandemic. In addition, 29% of respondents said they avoided information because it was untrustworthy or biased.

Information about the coronavirus is critical to controlling the pandemic but too much information may be counterproductive, resulting in the public's fatigue, overload, and avoidance of information. As we presented in Chapter 6, misinformation related to COVID-19-elicited negative emotions such as anxiety. Freiling et al. (2021) pointed out that anxiety causes people to be sensitive about pandemic information they encounter, which may further make them feel overwhelmed and overloaded.

Staying current about the pandemic situation is crucial for the well-being of the general public as well as the success of government mass vaccination campaigns. Unfortunately, the increase of information avoidance has been observed on the rise since the COVID-19 outbreak in various Western

DOI: 10.4324/9781003355984-9

countries, including the UK, Netherlands, and Norway (De Bruin et al., 2021; Kalogeropoulos et al., 2020; Ytre-Arne & Moe, 2021).

Therefore, into the third year of the global pandemic, what is the state of the public's information load in the four studied cities? Does the spread of misinformation surrounding COVID-19 make the problem worse? If so, how? More importantly, what is the consequence of information overload? Do respondents avoid COVID-19 information all together due to information overload? Using survey data collected from four parallel telephone surveys in August 2022, we examine these questions in this chapter.

Information Overload and Avoidance

Information overload refers to a perceptual state of feeling that the information one has received is overwhelming and too much to process (Jensen et al., 2020). That is, the amount of information available to an individual for viewing and processing is higher than his/her cognitive capacity (Eppler & Mengis, 2003). According to cognitive load theory (CLT), the human brain can only process a limited amount of information at a time (Apuke et al., 2022). Thus, information overload represents a type of cognitive load related to the excessive amount of information people receive, which puts burdens on their brains to process, evaluate, and act on the information.

In today's high-choice media environment, it is widely observed that an increasing number of people choose to avoid certain kinds of information (Palmer & Toff, 2020) or choose to tune out from mass media (De Bruin et al., 2021). Bawden and Robinson (2009) attributed information overload to exposure to large amounts of information from multiple channels, traditional and social media. Others have suggested a link between information overload and the quality of information. As Hong and Kim (2020) argued, the quality of information, rather than mere amount, is associated with uncertainty and ambiguity. Accordingly, information overload is not just a matter of information quantity but also a matter of information quality. When both factors are present, people have reported feelings of "too much."

The overload phenomenon is particularly pronounced in health-related information. In the context of infodemic, misinformation about the pandemic represents a type of low-quality misleading information during the initial COVID outbreaks worldwide. As we reported in Chapter 2, misinformation tends to be short, anonymous, and untraceable. Research has indicated that encounters with misinformation on social media through exposure or sharing contribute to peoples' cognitive load. As Islam et al. (2020) explained, a state of cognitive overload occurs when people are overwhelmed by the flux of information, leaving limited cognitive resources at their disposal. Hong and Kim (2020) reported that cognitive capacity and frequencies of news consumption and interpersonal communication about the COVID-19 pandemic were significantly related to information overload. Others (e.g.,

Mohammed et al., 2022) found a positive relationship between frequency of receiving COVID-19 information on social media and respondents' information overload in a number of countries.

According to Islam et al. (2020), "cognitive overload" gives rise to people's social media fatigue and hinders them from verifying online information they view or share. Information overload thus influences how people process information (Hong & Kim, 2020), leaning them toward greater heuristic processing (e.g., a mental short-cut approach to process new information for a quick result) and less systematic processing (e.g., thinking and comprehending new information). Most people may just choose to avoid any new information when overload occurs. In other words, when people feel overwhelmed by an ocean of information, their motivation to make sense of new information is reduced and social media fatigue increases, leading to information avoidance (Guo et al., 2020).

Information avoidance represents a choice that users make when navigating their information consumption with the multiple available options (Tandoc & Kim, 2022). The phenomenon of information avoidance has gained scholarly attention (Edgerly, 2021; Toff & Kalogeropoulos, 2020). A number of factors have been identified as predictors of avoidance, including the news negativity, low personal issue involvement, and information overload (Pentina & Tarafdar, 2014). The positive relationship between information overload and avoidance has been well explored in particular (e.g., Guo et al., 2020; Soroya et al., 2021); it provides the footing for our analyses of the negative effects of misinformation on respondents' feelings of information overload and their conscious decision to avoid information.

Because information overload is a mental state resulting from encounters with information of all sorts from various channels, we contextualized the information overload and avoidance to the infodemic during the COVID-19 pandemic. We adapted measures from past studies in health communication (e.g., Jensen et al., 2014) for the purpose of our own analyses. A 5-point Likert scale (1 = totally disagree, 5 = strongly agree) was used in respondents' responses to three items: (1) Considering my limited time to read, I face too much information/news about COVID-19 on social media, (2) I feel overloaded with the amount of information/news available on media about the pandemic, and (3) I receive more information/news about the pandemic on social media than I can process. The items were averaged to generate a measure of information overload ($M = 2.65$, $SD = 1.09$, $\alpha = .83$).

Similarly, our measurement of information avoidance was adapted from Miles et al. (2008), using the same 5-point Likert scale to measure respondents' agreement with these statements: (1) I prefer not to think about COVID-19, (2) I don't want any more information about COVID-19, and (3) I avoid learning about COVID-19. The average score formed the index of information avoidance ($M = 2.23$, $SD = 1.01$, $\alpha = .83$).

Findings

We performed a series of *t*-tests, followed by regression analyses, to explore who were mostly overloaded by information about COVID-19, who were likely to avoid information, and what individual- and macro-level factors might contribute to the avoidance behavior.

First, frequency analyses indicated that the respondents in the four cities seemed to tire of information about COVID-19 after enduring the pandemic for almost three years. Among the 4,094 respondents interviewed by telephone in August 2022, 25.4%–34.9% "agreed" and "strongly agreed" with the statement "Considering my limited time to read, I face too much information/news about COVID-19 on social media." In addition, 17.0% and 23.7% of the respondents "agreed" and "strongly agreed" that "I prefer not to think about COVID-19."

Demographics and Information Overload

To examine how respondents' information overload varied by their key demographics, we created subgroups by gender and age. Table 9.1 shows the gender difference in information overload. Male respondents ($M = 2.70$, $SD = 1.13$) were more overloaded than were female respondents ($M = 2.61$, $SD = 1.04$). The difference was statistically significant ($t = 2.58$, $p < .05$).

To measure the relationship of age and overload, we created a younger group (respondents from 18 to 46 years old; $n = 1,974$) and an older group (47–94 years old; $n = 2,177$). Older adults ($M = 2.70$, $SD = 1.13$) reported a higher level of information overload than did younger adults ($M = 2.61$, $SD = 1.04$) and the difference was significant (see Table 9.2 for details). These results confirm that age and gender matter regarding information overload.

Table 9.1 Gender differences in information overload during the COVID-19 pandemic

	Male (n = 2,006)	Female (n = 2,102)	
	M (SD)	M (SD)	t value
1 Considering my limited time to read, I face too much news on social media	2.94 (1.24)	2.86 (1.21)	2.02*
2 I feel overloaded with the amount of news available on media	2.58 (1.28)	2.49 (1.25)	2.39*
3 I receive more news than I can process on social media	2.59 (1.32)	2.49 (1.28)	2.38*
Combined index	2.70 (1.11)	2.61 (1.07)	2.58*

Note: The items were rated from 1 to 5, where 1 = totally disagree and 5 = strongly agree; *p < .05.

Information Exposure and Information Overload

To examine the relationship between information exposure and overload, respondents were differentiated into low (n = 1,925) and high (n = 2,129) information-exposure groups by splitting the scale at the median (refer to Chapter 4 for detailed measures). Exposure to COVID-19 information was measured by the averaged frequency score on three kinds of COVID-19 information with a 5-point scale: (1) information about vaccine effects on COVID-19, (2) information about COVID-19 prevention, and (3) information concerning how to fight the pandemic. As shown in Table 9.3, respondents with high (M = 2.62, SD = 1.12) and low (M = 2.69, SD = 1.05) COVID-19 information exposure exhibited different levels of information overload (t = 2.09, p < .05).

Table 9.2 Differences in information overload during the COVID-19 pandemic between older and younger adults

	Younger adults (n = 1,974)	Older adults (n = 2,117)	
	M (SD)	M (SD)	t value
1 Considering my limited time to read, I face too much news on social media	2.89 (1.15)	2.91 (1.30)	.64
2 I feel overloaded with the amount of news available on media	2.47 (1.26)	2.59 (1.31)	3.13**
3 I receive more news than I can process on social media	2.46 (1.26)	2.61 (1.33)	3.71***
Combined index	2.61 (1.04)	2.70 (1.13)	-2.91**

Note: The items were rated from 1 to 5, where 1 = totally disagree and 5 = strongly agree; **p < .01, ***p < .001.

Table 9.3 Differences in information overload during the COVID-19 pandemic between individuals of low and high COVID-19 information exposure

	Low information exposure (n = 1,925)	High information exposure (n = 2,129)	
	M (SD)	M (SD)	t value
1 Considering my limited time to read, I face too much news on social media	2.89 (1.17)	2.90 (1.28)	–.33
2 I feel overloaded with the amount of news available on media	2.59 (1.23)	2.48 (1.29)	2.94**
3 I receive more news than I can process on social media	2.59 (1.26)	2.49 (1.34)	2.59*
Combined index	2.69 (1.05)	2.62 (1.12)	2.09*

Note: The items were rated from 1 to 5, where 1 = totally disagree and 5 = strongly agree; *p < .05, **p < .01.

Misinformation Exposure and Information Overload

To further explore the relationship between exposure to COVID-19 misinformation and information overload, we divided the respondents into groups of low (n = 2,067) and high misinformation exposure (n = 1,849) and compared their information-overload perception. As shown in Table 9.4, respondents who had less misinformation exposure (M = 2.50, SD = 1.03) were less overloaded (t = –9.95, p < .001) compared to respondents who were exposed more to misinformation about COVID-19 (M = 2.84, SD = 1.12). These results suggest that exposure to misinformation about the pandemic was related to the mental state of overload.

Misinformation Beliefs and Information Overloaded

To explore how misbelief is related to information overload, we distinguished high- (n = 2,027) and low-misbelief (n = 1,966) respondents by splitting the scale at the median (Chapter 8 provides the measurement). As shown in Table 9.5, respondents who had more misbeliefs about COVID-19 (M = 2.78, SD = 1.06) reported a higher level of information overload, compared to those who had less misbeliefs (M = 2.50, SD = 1.11). The difference was statistically significant (t = –8.19, p < .001).

Anti-Vaccine Attitudes and Information Overload

We also analyzed the relationship between anti-vaccine attitudes and information overload by dividing the respondents into groups of low (n = 2,178) and high (n = 1,902) anti-vaccine attitudes (splitting the scale at the median;

Table 9.4 Differences in information overload during the COVID-19 pandemic between individuals of low and high level of exposure to COVID-19 misinformation

	Low misinformation exposure (n = 2,067)	High misinformation exposure (n = 1,849)	
	M (SD)	M (SD)	t value
1 Considering my limited time to read, I face too much news on social media	2.74 (1.19)	3.09 (1.24)	–9.00***
2 I feel overloaded with the amount of news available on media	2.37 (1.20)	2.71 (1.31)	–8.37***
3 I receive more news than I can process on social media	2.37 (1.23)	2.72 (1.35)	–8.37***
Combined index	2.50 (1.03)	2.84 (1.12)	–9.95***

Note: The items were rated from 1 to 5, where 1 = totally disagree and 5 = strongly agree; ***p < .001.

Table 9.5 Differences in information overload during the COVID-19 pandemic between individuals of low and high level of beliefs in COVID-19 misinformation

	Low beliefs (n = 1,966)	High beliefs (n = 2,027)	
	M (SD)	M (SD)	t value
1 Considering my limited time to read, I face too much news on social media	2.78 (1.25)	3.01 (1.20)	−5.88***
2 I feel overloaded with the amount of news available on media	2.37 (1.26)	2.67 (1.25)	−7.34***
3 I receive more news than I can process on social media	2.37 (1.29)	2.69 (1.29)	−7.84***
Combined index	2.50 (1.11)	2.78 (1.06)	−8.19***

Note: The items were rated from 1 to 5, where 1 = totally disagree and 5 = strongly agree; ***$p < .001$.

Table 9.6 Differences in information overload during the COVID-19 pandemic between individuals of low and high level of anti-vaccine attitude

	Low anti-vaccine attitude (n = 2,178)	High anti-vaccine attitude (n = 1,902)	
	M (SD)	M (SD)	t value
1 Considering my limited time to read, I face too much news on social media	2.63 (1.22)	3.21 (1.16)	−15.70***
2 I feel overloaded with the amount of news available on media	2.20 (1.17)	2.91 (1.26)	−18.67***
3 I receive more news than I can process on social media	2.19 (1.21)	2.93 (1.29)	−18.92***
Combined index	2.34 (1.01)	3.02 (1.06)	−2.89***

Note: The items were rated from 1 to 5, where 1 = totally disagree and 5 = strongly agree; ***$p < .001$.

the detailed measurement is found in Chapter 7). As shown in Table 9.6, significant differences existed between the two groups. Compared to respondents who had a higher level of anti-vaccine attitudes ($M = 3.02$, $SD = 1.061$), those who had lower anti-vaccine attitudes were less overloaded ($M = 2.34$, $SD = 1.01$), $t = −2.89$, $p < .001$.

Risk Acceptance and Information Overload

To explore if risk acceptance and information overload were related, we divided the scale of risk acceptance at the median to separate respondents into high-risk-acceptance ($n = 2,288$) and low-risk-acceptance ($n = 1,793$)

Table 9.7 Differences in information overload during the COVID-19 pandemic between individuals of low and high level of risk acceptance

	Low risk acceptance (n = 1,793)	High risk acceptance (n = 2,288)	
	M (SD)	M (SD)	t value
1 Considering my limited time to read, I face too much news on social media	2.81 (1.19)	2.97 (1.24)	–2.64**
2 I feel overloaded with the amount of news available on media	2.45 (1.21)	2.60 (1.30)	–3.33**
3 I receive more news than I can process on social media	2.41 (1.24)	2.64 (1.34)	–6.25***
Combined index	2.55 (1.04)	2.74 (1.12)	–4.70***

Note: The items were rated from 1 to 5, where 1 = totally disagree and 5 = strongly agree; ***$p < .001$.

groups. Risk acceptance was measured by agreements on three items with a 5-point scale: (1) I believe I have high acceptance of potential risks engendered by the spread of COVID-19, (2) I believe I can bear with the risk of living with COVID-19, and (3) I believe I can accept the potential risks brought by COVID-19 infection on my health. As shown in Table 9.7, respondents who had a lower level of risk acceptance ($M = 2.55$, $SD = 1.04$) were less overloaded, compared to those who had a higher level of risk acceptance ($M = 2.74$, $SD = 1.12$), $t = -4.70$, $p < .001$. This particular result indicates that respondents who felt less comfortable accepting COVID-19 as a risk to live with were less burned by information about the pandemic.

Cross-City Differences in Information Overload

We compared the differences in information overload among respondents from Beijing ($n = 1,033$), Hong Kong ($n = 1,017$), Taipei ($n = 1,019$), and Singapore ($n = 1,025$) to explore if living with different pandemic-control policies would affect information overload. Based on the results in Table 9.8, cross-city differences were found. Respondents in Singapore perceived a higher level of information overload ($M = 3.25$, $SD = .91$) than their counterparts in the other three cities (Beijing ($M = 2.57$, $SD = 1.01$), Taipei ($M = 2.51$, $SD = 1.10$), and Hong Kong ($M = 2.27$, $SD = 1.06$). ANOVA testing showed the difference in information overload among four cities was significant, $F(3, 4098) = 175.33$, $p < .001$.

Table 9.8 Differences in information overload during the COVID-19 pandemic across Beijing, Hong Kong, Taipei, and Singapore

	Beijing (n = 1,033)	Hong Kong (n = 1,017)	Taipei (n = 1,019)	Singapore (n = 1,025)	Total	F value
1 Considering my limited time to read, I face too much news on social media	2.47 (1.20)	2.14 (1.23)	2.36 (1.24)	3.13 (1.16)	3.21 (1.16)	127.04***
2 I feel overloaded with the amount of news available on media	2.92 (1.18)	2.46 (1.24)	2.75 (1.30)	3.44 (.96)	3.50 (1.21)	127.95***
3 I receive more news than I can process on social media	2.31 (1.19)	2.20 (1.29)	2.43 (1.29)	3.18 (1.20)	3.48 (1.22)	130.71***
Combined index	2.57 (1.01)	2.27 (1.06)	2.51 (1.10)	3.25 (.91)	3.40 (1.08)	175.33***

Note: The items were rated from 1 to 5, where 1 = totally disagree and 5 = strongly agree; ***$p < .001$.

Predictors of Information Overload

We ran hierarchical regression analyses to examine the effects of demographics, information exposure, misinformation exposure, misbeliefs, anti-vaccine attitudes, and risk acceptance on information overload. As shown in Table 9.9, age ($\beta = .06$, $p < .01$) and gender ($\beta = .04$, $p < .01$) were significant predictors of information overload. Education was negatively correlated with information overload ($\beta = -.10$, $p < .001$), suggesting that those who were more educated were less overloaded. Respondents in Beijing were not different from respondents in other three cities in terms of overloaded ($\beta = .03$, $p > .05$).

Controlling for the influences of the demographics, information exposure was not significantly related with information overload ($\beta = .00$, $p > .05$). But exposure to misinformation was positively correlated with information overload ($\beta = .12$, $p < .001$). Misbeliefs were not significantly correlated with information overload ($\beta = .02$, $p > .05$). Other significant and positive predictors were: higher levels of anti-vaccine attitude ($\beta = .32$, $p < .001$) and risk acceptance of living with COVID ($\beta = .07$, $p < .001$). Together, these predictors explained 16.0% of the variance in the level of information overload, suggesting that respondents who had stronger anti-vaccine attitudes and those with a higher level of comfort of living with COVID as a risk were more overwhelmed.

Table 9.9 Hierarchical regression analysis predicting information overload during the COVID-19 pandemic

Predictors	Information overload
Block 1: Demographics	
Age	.06**
Gender (Male = 1)	.04**
Education	−.10***
City (Beijing = 1)	.03
Adjusted R^2	1.7%
Block 2: Information exposure	
Information exposure	.00
Incremental adjusted R^2	0.0%
Block 3: Misinformation exposure	
Misinformation exposure	.12***
Incremental adjusted R^2	3.6%
Block 4: Misinformation beliefs	
Misinformation beliefs	.02
Incremental adjusted R^2	1.9%
Block 5: Anti-vaccine attitude	
Anti-vaccine attitude	.32***
Incremental adjusted R^2	8.4%
Block 6: Risk acceptance	
Risk acceptance	.07***
Incremental adjusted R^2	0.4%
Total adjusted R^2	16.0%

Note: $N = 3,741$; **$p < .01$, ***$p < .001$.

Demographic Patterns of Information Avoidance

In the rest of this chapter, we explored the patterns of information avoidance. As Table 9.10 shows, male respondents ($M = 2.32$, $SD = 1.14$) had a higher level of information avoidance than did female respondents ($M = 2.20$, $SD = 1.07$); the difference was statistically significant ($t = 3.33$, $p < .001$). Table 9.11 shows that younger adults ($M = 2.23$, $SD = 1.06$) had a slightly lower level of information avoidance than older adults did ($M = 2.29$, $SD = 1.15$). The difference was significant ($t = -1.89$, $p < .05$). Based on these results, the tendency to avoid information about COVID-19 is related to gender and age.

Information Exposure and Information Avoidance

To examine if information avoidance varied by frequency of information exposure, we used the median to divide the respondents into groups of low ($n = 1,926$) and high information exposure ($n = 2,123$; the n changed slightly due to missing values). The results of independent t-tests presented

Table 9.10 Gender differences in information avoidance during the COVID-19 pandemic

	Male (n = 2,006)	Female (n = 2,103)	
	M (SD)	M (SD)	t value
1 I don't want any more information about COVID-19	2.40 (1.31)	2.27 (1.22)	3.32**
2 I avoid learning about COVID-19	2.16 (1.30)	2.03 (1.21)	3.23**
3 I prefer not to think about COVID-19	2.40 (1.36)	2.31 (1.29)	2.10*
Combined index	2.32 (1.14)	2.20 (1.07)	3.33**

Note: The items were rated from 1 to 5, where 1 = totally disagree and 5 = strongly agree; $**p < .01$, $***p < .001$.

Table 9.11 Differences in information avoidance during the COVID-19 pandemic between younger and older adults

	Younger adults (n = 1,975)	Older adults (n = 2,119)	
	M (SD)	M (SD)	t value
1 I don't want any more information about COVID-19	2.28 (1.22)	2.39 (1.31)	−2.78**
2 I avoid learning about COVID-19	2.05 (1.22)	2.14 (1.29)	−2.42*
3 I prefer not to think about COVID-19	2.36 (1.30)	2.35 (1.35)	.23
Combined index	2.23 (1.06)	2.29 (1.15)	−1.89*

Note: The items were rated from 1 to 5, where 1 = totally disagree and 5 = strongly agree; $*p < .05$, $**p < .01$.

in Table 9.12 show that respondents with low-level information exposure exhibited a higher level of information avoidance (M = 2.48, SD = 1.12) than those with a high level of information exposure (M = 2.05, SD = 1.05). The difference was significant (t = 12.65, p < .001).

Misinformation Exposure and Information Avoidance

To investigate if information avoidance was related to misinformation exposure, we separated the respondents into groups of high (n = 1,852) and low misinformation exposure (n = 2,069) by median of the scale. As Table 9.13 shows, respondents of low misinformation exposure (M = 2.25, SD = 1.10) did not differ in information avoidance from those of high misinformation exposure (M = 2.27, SD = 1.12), t = −.70, p > .05. That is, the level of exposure to misinformation about COVID-19 was not related to tendency to avoid information.

Table 9.12 Differences in information avoidance during the COVID-19 pandemic between individuals of low and high level of COVID-19 information exposure

	Low information exposure (n = 1,926)	High information exposure (n = 2,123)	
	M (SD)	M (SD)	t value
1 I don't want any more information about COVID-19	2.54 (1.28)	2.14 (1.22)	10.05***
2 I avoid learning about COVID-19	2.30 (1.30)	1.89 (1.18)	10.59***
3 I prefer not to think about COVID-19	2.61 (1.34)	2.12 (1.27)	11.95***
Combined index	2.48 (1.12)	2.05 (1.05)	12.65***

Note: The items were rated from 1 to 5, where 1 = totally disagree and 5 = strongly agree; ***$p < .001$.

Table 9.13 Differences in information avoidance during the COVID-19 pandemic between individuals of low and high level of exposure to COVID-19 misinformation

	Low misinformation exposure (n = 2,069)	High misinformation exposure (n = 1,852)	
	M (SD)	M (SD)	t value
1 I don't want any more information about COVID-19	2.30 (1.25)	2.37 (1.29)	−1.81
2 I avoid learning about COVID-19	2.11 (1.25)	2.08 (1.26)	.78
3 I prefer not to think about COVID-19	2.34 (1.31)	2.37 (1.34)	−.75
Combined index	2.25 (1.10)	2.27 (1.12)	−.70

Note: The items were rated from 1 to 5, where 1 = totally disagree and 5 = strongly agree.

Misbeliefs and Information Avoidance

We further examined if level of information avoidance differed between respondents with different levels of misbeliefs about COVID-19. We categorized the respondents into two groups based on the median of misinformation beliefs scale. Table 9.14 showed that respondents who believed in misinformation less tended to avoid information less ($M = 2.08$, $SD = 1.06$) than did those with a higher level of misbeliefs ($M = 2.43$, $SD = 1.13$), $t = −9.99$, $p < .001$.

Anti-Vaccine Attitudes and Information Avoidance

We also compared differences in information avoidance between respondents who held weak (n = 2,182) and strong anti-vaccine attitudes (n = 1,904). Results in Table 9.15 indicated a significant difference (t = –18.29, p < .001). Respondents who had a lower level of anti-vaccine attitudes (M = 1.97, SD = 1.01) tended to avoid information less than those who had a higher level of anti-vaccine attitudes (M = 2.59, SD = 1.12).

Table 9.14 Differences in information avoidance during the COVID-19 pandemic between individuals of low and high level of beliefs in COVID-19 misinformation

	Low beliefs (n = 1,972)	High beliefs (n = 2,028)	
	M (SD)	M (SD)	t value
1 I don't want any more information about COVID-19	2.17 (1.22)	2.48 (1.29)	–7.79***
2 I avoid learning about COVID-19	1.92 (1.20)	2.26 (1.29)	–8.48***
3 I prefer not to think about COVID-19	2.15 (1.28)	2.54 (1.34)	–9.54***
Combined index	2.08 (1.06)	2.43 (1.13)	–9.99***

Note: The items were rated from 1 to 5, where 1 = totally disagree and 5 = strongly agree; ***p < .001.

Table 9.15 Differences in information avoidance during the COVID-19 pandemic between individuals of low and high level of anti-vaccine attitudes

	Low anti-vaccine attitude (n = 2,182)	High anti-vaccine attitude (n = 1,904)	
	M (SD)	M (SD)	t value
1 I don't want any more information about COVID-19	2.06 (1.19)	2.65 (1.28)	–15.19***
2 I avoid learning about COVID-19	1.83 (1.14)	2.39 (1.31)	–14.33***
3 I prefer not to think about COVID-19	2.02 (1.20)	2.73 (1.36)	–17.37***
Combined index	1.97 (1.01)	2.59 (1.12)	–18.29***

Note: The items were rated from 1 to 5, where 1 = totally disagree and 5 = strongly agree; ***p < .001.

Risk Acceptance and Information Avoidance

To examine how risk acceptance was related to information avoidance, we next divided the respondents into the low-risk-acceptance (n = 1,678) and high-risk acceptance (n = 2,416) groups. The *t*-test results showed no significant difference (t = −.45, p > .05). Respondents who had a higher level of risk acceptance of living with COVID-19 (M = 2.51, SD = 1.21) and those who had a lower level of risk acceptance (M = 2.49, SD = .90) seemed to have a similar tendency to avoid information.

Cross-City Differences in Information Avoidance

By running a series of ANOVA tests, we found a significant difference [F(3, 4105) = 9.97, p < .001] in information avoidance among respondents in Beijing (n = 1,033), Hong Kong (n = 1,017), Taipei (n = 1,019), and Singapore (n = 1,025). As results in Table 9.16 show, compared to respondents in Beijing (M = 2.29, SD = 1.11), Singapore (M = 2.24, SD = .95), and Taipei (M = 2.13, SD = 1.09), respondents in Hong Kong had a higher level of information avoidance (M = 2.39, SD = 1.24).

Predictors of Information Avoidance

Hierarchical regression analyses examined the effects of the key variables (e.g., demographics, information exposure, misinformation exposure, misinformation beliefs, anti-vaccine attitude, and risk acceptance) on information

Table 9.16 Differences in information avoidance during the COVID-19 pandemic across Beijing, Hong Kong, Taipei, and Singapore

	Beijing (n = 1,033)	Hong Kong (n = 1,017)	Taipei (n = 1,019)	Singapore (n = 1,025)	Total	F value
1 I don't want any more information about COVID-19	2.45 (1.24)	2.38 (1.41)	2.24 (1.25)	2.27 (1.14)	2.48 (1.18)	6.33***
2 I avoid learning about COVID-19	2.16 (1.28)	2.28 (1.43)	1.99 (1.19)	1.96 (1.07)	2.47 (1.20)	15.25***
3 I prefer not to think about COVID-19	2.27 (1.26)	2.50 (1.42)	2.15 (1.27)	2.50 (1.31)	2.56 (1.22)	18.08***
Combined index	2.29 (1.11)	2.39 (1.24)	2.13 (1.09)	2.24 (0.95)	2.50 (1.10)	9.97***

Note: The items were rated from 1 to 5, where 1 = totally disagree and 5 = strongly agree; ***p < .001.

Table 9.17 Hierarchical regression analysis predicting information avoidance during the COVID-19 pandemic

Predictors	Information avoidance
Block 1: Demographics	
Age	.04**
Gender (Male = 1)	.04**
Education	−.09***
City (Beijing = 1)	.08***
Adjusted R²	3.2%
Block 2: Information exposure	
Information exposure	−.19***
Incremental adjusted R²	4.7%
Block 3: Misinformation exposure	
Misinformation exposure	−.03***
Incremental adjusted R²	0.6%
Block 4: Misinformation beliefs	
Misinformation beliefs	.02
Incremental adjusted R²	1.8%
Block 5: Anti-vaccine attitude	
Anti-vaccine attitude	.17***
Incremental adjusted R²	7.1%
Block 6: Risk acceptance	
Risk acceptance	.07***
Incremental adjusted R²	0.8%
Block 7: Information overload	
Overload	.38***
Incremental adjusted R²	11.7%
Total adjusted R²	29.9%

Note: N = 3,746; ***$p < .001$.

avoidance. Results in Table 9.17 show that education was negatively related to information avoidance (β = −.09, $p < .001$), suggesting that respondents with a higher education level tended to avoid information less. Older respondents were more likely to avoid information compared to younger ones (β = .04, $p < .01$). Male respondents were more likely to avoid information compared to females (β = .04, $p < .01$).

In addition to demographic predictors, information exposure (β = −.19, $p < .001$) and misinformation exposure (β = −.03, $p < .001$) were negative predictors of information avoidance. Moreover, respondents who held a higher level of anti-vaccine attitudes tended to avoid information more (β = .17, $p < .001$). So did those with a higher level of risk acceptance on living with COVID-19 (β = .07, $p < .001$). Additionally, information overload was a positive predictor of avoidance (β = .38, $p < .001$). In fact, it was the strongest among the predictors, indicating a dependable relationship between overload and avoidance. When the information about COVID-19 became too much, respondents quit.

Together, these predictors explained 29.9% of the variance in frequency of information avoidance, which indicates that respondents who encountered misinformation more frequently, had more misbeliefs in misinformation, held stronger anti-vaccine attitudes, and experienced greater acceptance of living with COVID-19 tended to avoid information more.

Summary of Key Findings

The key findings from the telephone surveys in the four cities of this chapter can be summarized into general patterns in information overload and intention to avoid information about COVID-19:

- In terms of demographics, male respondents felt more overloaded than did their female counterparts. Older adults felt more overloaded than did younger adults. Further, male respondents had a higher level of avoidance than did female respondents. Older adults had a higher level of avoidance than did younger adults.
- Respondents who were exposed more to COVID-19 information felt less overloaded than those who were exposed less to such information. Moreover, those who were exposed more to COVID-19 misinformation felt more overloaded than did those who were exposed less. Regarding information avoidance, those who encountered COVID-19 information more had a lower level of avoidance.
- Those who held more misbeliefs were more overloaded than those who believed less. But they had a higher level of avoidance. Respondents with a higher level of anti-vaccine attitudes felt more overloaded than did those with a lower level of anti-vaccine attitude. They had a higher level of avoidance than those who had a lower level of anti-vaccine attitude.
- Respondents felt more overloaded when they had a higher level of risk acceptance and reported a higher level of avoidance.
- Respondents in Singapore, with its living with COVID policy, felt the most overloaded, followed by respondents in Beijing, Taipei, and Hong Kong. In terms of information avoidance, respondents in Hong Kong had the highest level of avoidance, followed by respondents in Beijing, Singapore, and Taipei.
- When all factors are considered together, those that account for the differences in information overload are age, gender, education, misinformation exposure, anti-vaccine attitude, and risk acceptance. Factors that account for the differences in information avoidance are age, gender, education, place of residence, information exposure, misinformation exposure, anti-vaccine attitude, risk acceptance, and information overload.

Qualitative Findings

Information as a Burden

When there's overwhelming COVID-19-related information online and offline, participants need to invest more time and energy if they wish to understand and evaluate the contents; processing tons of COVID-19-related information risks overload. The account from Elijah, a Hong Kong male student, is revealing; he told his focus group that he muted his family's group chat because there was too much information on a daily basis. He called this "pandemic fatigue."

A 58-year-old male accounting manager Benjamin also living in Hong Kong disclosed that he spends up to seven hours on social media every day because he always follows COVID-19-related information. He admitted that he feels overwhelmed by loads of information. "The information from the Department of Health is reliable," he explained.

> I wouldn't say so for other information sources because some of them are just passing false messages. Even on YouTube, you can find a lot of information about this pandemic, and the question remains whether you should believe it or not. There's too much different information, and you can't read it all. Others forward too many messages and you cannot get updated on the most precise one. If there's something I really want to know, I will go to the website of the Department of Health to see whether they have some information there.

Participants disclosed that information overload may cause them to avoid seeking COVID-19-related information just to get their lives back. A 22-year-old female participant in Beijing Ms. Liu said that she quit using several social media platforms because she found too much misinformation on them. She continued,

> I don't think any of the platforms are reliable. I used to rely on Weibo, but then I found people always sending out suspicious messages. Then I followed the information on Red Book, and they did similar things there. Gradually, I gave up on those platforms. Now, when someone tells me that there are [confirmed cases] here and there, well, I will take it as what it is.

Similarly, a 44-year-old male participant Mateo in Singapore decided to quit social media after he found out the messages there are misleading. In his words,

> After a few incidents or events, I stopped going to social media, just like in the first year of COVID or the second year of COVID, Vietnam is reporting that they are the safest area. They don't need any quarantine. The number of people infected is below thousands or below about 5,000,

which is for a population of millions in one city. It is very, very, very low. So, people think that it is a very safe place. But when I go there and talk to my colleagues and client there, everybody is falling sick.

Some participants indicated that because of overload they intended to receive information from health authorities as verified information from a reliable source. A 50-year-old female sales manager Sofia in Singapore said that she "doesn't believe in social media at all because there is a lot of fake news out there." Instead, she consults the Ministry of Health for essential information. A younger male participant in Singapore Alexander also tended to follow verified sources and believed that he would learn about important information: "When it's really breaking news or like huge news, it will just somehow appear on your iPhone as a notification."

Cross-City Differences

Participants in Hong Kong, where the highest level of COVID-19-related information avoidance was recorded, avoided related information with disappointment and dissatisfaction. A 52-year-old female participant Mia in Hong Kong said,

I'll take a glance at the titles of notifications from news apps on my phone. But if the contents are about numbers such as how many people are infected and how many people die every day, I have no interest in reading it, thinking why these again? I'll clear all these messages immediately when there are notifications. I don't take a look at them at all. What do you want me to think of or react to these numbers? There's been no improvement for the past two years, so why tell me the numbers? It's useless and not helpful to me.

William, a 49-year-old male engineer in Hong Kong chimed in,

It's a sort of numbness... The director of the Department of Health, the Chief Executive... They always say Hong Kong will not take the 'lying flat' (do nothing) approach, but the new policies definitely show a trend toward 'lying flat'. I feel that they say something and do another. So, the information is not so useful.

With COVID policy relaxing, a 54-year-old male engineer in Singapore Jackson disclosed that he stopped following COVID-19-related information. He explained,

I feel that one day... do you think that are you able to control the coronavirus situation now? I feel not really; otherwise, how come the news will report how many cases we have every day? That means it's not under control, but the severity is not high, so it should be OK.

Living with strict restrictions under zero-COVID policy in Beijing, Ms. Hu, a 45-year-old female participant working in finance, revealed that she avoided COVID-19-related information for a different reason: The expectation of going back to normal life. She said,

> When the pandemic had just started two years ago, we were nervous, and we would keep talking about it at that time. But now we're all tired of it. We don't talk about it anymore. We talk about something else. We just want to get our lives back to normal. We still need to wear masks, display Health Kit (*Jian Kang Bao*), and do PCR tests, all of these are counted as annoyances, and not welcomed. So we don't talk about the pandemic anymore. Instead, we talk about something more light-hearted.

Insights and Implications for Public Policy

Considering that being informed about the pandemic situation with sufficient updated and scientific information is crucial for public health and successful pandemic control, a few insights can be drawn from the findings of this chapter.

First, public health authorities need to pay attention to the issue of "too much" information about the pandemic, especially among older people and women. Too much information causes overload for them. Misinformation tends to worsen the problem. It also motivates citizens to avoid information altogether. Thus, the government needs to do more to ensure timely and factually correct information is available to the public as the pandemic persists.

Second, because information overload causes the intention to avoid information, more information would be counterproductive. To keep the public informed, public institutions involved in the prevention and control of pandemics need to consider setting a limit in the amount of information they send out for public consumption.

Finally, in societies such as Singapore that have adopted a living with COVID policy, the issue of too much information appears to be particularly burdensome to their residents. Public health agencies need to monitor their updates and daily briefings carefully to avoid a tipping point of swamping their citizens with more information than they can handle.

References

Apuke, O. D., Omar, B., Tunca, E. A., & Gever, C. V. (2022). Information overload and misinformation sharing behaviour of social media users: Testing the moderating role of cognitive ability. *Journal of Information Science*. https://doi.org/10.1177/01655515221121942

Bawden, D., & Robinson, L. (2009). The dark side of information: Overload, anxiety and other paradoxes and pathologies. *Journal of Information Science, 35*(2), 180–191. https://doi.org/10.1177/0165551508095781

De Bruin, K., de Haan, Y., Vliegenthart, R., Kruikemeier, S., & Boukes, M. (2021). News avoidance during the COVID-19 crisis: Understanding information overload. *Digital Journalism, 9*(9), 1286–1302. https://doi.org/10.1080/21670811.20 21.1957967

Edgerly, S. (2021). The head and heart of news avoidance: How attitudes about the news media relate to levels of news consumption. *Journalism, 23*(9), 1828–1845 https://doi.org/10.1177/14648849211012922

Eppler, M. J., & Mengis, J. (2003). A framework for information overload research in organizations. *Università della Svizzera italiana, 2003*.

Freiling, I., Krause, N. M., Scheufele, D. A., & Brossard, D. (2021). Believing and sharing misinformation, fact-checks, and accurate information on social media: The role of anxiety during COVID-19. *New Media & Society*. https://doi. org/10.1177/14614448211011451

Guo, Y., Lu, Z., Kuang, H., & Wang, C. (2020). Information avoidance behavior on social network sites: Information irrelevance, overload, and the moderating role of time pressure. *International Journal of Information Management, 52*. https://doi. org/10.1016/j.ijinfomgt.2020.102067

Hong, H., & Kim, H. J. (2020). Antecedents and consequences of information overload in the COVID-19 pandemic. *International Journal of Environmental Research and Public Health, 17*(24), 9305. https://doi.org/10.3390/ijerph17249305

Islam, A. K. M. N., Laato, S., Talukder, S., & Sutinen, E. (2020). Misinformation sharing and social media fatigue during COVID-19: An affordance and cognitive load perspective. *Technological Forecasting and Social Change, 159*, 120201. https://doi.org/10.1016/j.techfore.2020.120201

Jensen, J. D., Carcioppolo, N., King, A. J., Scherr, C. L., Jones, C. L., & Niederdeppe, J. (2014). The cancer information overload (CIO) scale: Establishing predictive and discriminant validity. *Patient Education and Counseling, 94*(1), 90–96. https://doi. org/10.1016/j.pec.2013.09.016

Jensen, J. D., Pokharel, M., Carcioppolo, N., Upshaw, S., John, K. K., & Katz, R. A. (2020). Cancer information overload: Discriminant validity and relationship to sun safe behaviors. *Patient Education and Counseling, 103*(2), 309–314. https://doi. org/10.1016/j.pec.2019.08.039

Kalogeropoulos, A., Fletcher, R., & Nielsen, R. K. (2020). *Initial surge in news use around Coronavirus in the UK has been followed by significant increase in news avoidance*. Reuters Institute for the Study of Journalism. https://reutersinstitute. politics.ox.ac.uk/initial-surge-news-use-around-coronavirus-uk-has-been-followed-significant-increase-news-avoidance

Miles, A., Voorwinden, S., Chapman, S., & Wardle, J. (2008). Psychologic predictors of cancer information avoidance among older adults: The role of cancer fear and fatalism. *Cancer Epidemiology and Prevention Biomarkers, 17*(8), 1872–1879. https://doi.org/10.1158/1055-9965.EPI-08-0074

Mohammed, M., Sha'aban, A., Jatau, A. I., Yunusa, I., Isa, A. M., Wada, A. S., Obamiro, K., Zainal, H., & Ibrahim, B. (2022). Assessment of COVID-19 information overload among the general public. *Journal of Racial and Ethnic Health Disparities, 9*(1), 184–192. https://doi.org/10.1007/s40615-020-00942-0

Newman, N., Fletcher, R., Kalogeropoulos, A., Levy, D., & Nielsen, R. K. (2017). *Reuters Institute Digital News Report 2017*. Oxford: Reuters Institute for the Study of Journalism. https://www.digitalnewsreport.org/survey/2017/

Newman, N., Fletcher, R., Roberson, C. T., Eddy, K., & Nielsen, R. K. (2022). *Reuters Institute Digital News Report 2022*. Oxford: Reuters Institute for the Study of Journalism. https://reutersinstitute.politics.ox.ac.uk/digital-news-report/2022

Palmer, R., & Toff, B. (2020). What does it take to sustain a news habit? The role of civic duty norms and a connection to a "news community" among news avoiders in the UK and Spain. *International Journal of Communication, 14*, 1634–1653. https://ijoc.org/index.php/ijoc/article/view/12252

Pentina, I., & Tarafdar, M. (2014). From "information" to "knowing": Exploring the role of social media in contemporary news consumption. *Computers in Human Behavior, 35*, 211–223. https://doi.org/10.1016/j.chb.2014.02.045

Soroya, S. H., Farooq, A., Mahmood, K., Isoaho, J., & Zara, S. E. (2021). From information seeking to information avoidance: Understanding the health information behavior during a global health crisis. *Information Processing & Management, 58*(2). https://doi.org/10.1016/j.ipm.2020.102440

Tandoc, Jr., E. C., & Kim, H. K. (2022). Avoiding real news, believing in fake news? Investigating pathways from information overload to misbelief. *Journalism*. https://doi.org/10.1177/14648849221090744

Toff, B., & Kalogeropoulos, A. (2020). All the news that's fit to ignore: How the information environment does and does not shape news avoidance. *Public Opinion Quarterly, 84*(S1), 366–390. https://doi.org/10.1093/poq/nfaa016

Ytre-Arne, B., & Moe, H. (2021). Doomscrolling, monitoring and avoiding: News use in COVID-19 pandemic Lockdown. *Journalism Studies, 22*(13), 1739–1755. https://doi.org/10.1080/1461670X.2021.1952475

10 Fighting Back

Citizen Actions to Combat Misinformation

Dong Dong, Grace Xiao Zhang, and Yan Zeng

Introduction

Their geographical proximity to the COVID-19 epicenter, Wuhan, China, makes the cities of Beijing, Hong Kong, Singapore, and Taiwan the first to be hit by the pandemic and the infodemic. As presented in the previous four chapters, encountering misinformation surrounding COVID-19 on social media adversely affects citizens in the four cities, ranging from eliciting negative emotions and biased risk perception (Chapter 6), forming anti-vaccine attitudes (Chapter 7), acceptance of misbeliefs and hindering knowledge gain about the pandemic (Chapter 8), and information overload during the pandemic (Chapter 9). A number of pressing questions arose from these key findings: How do respondents cope with misinformation about COVID-19 on social media? To what extent does the general public support government actions to restrict misinformation? For citizens, what actions do they take to combat misinformation?

In fact, since the emergence of rumors and misinformation about the pandemic, the public has engaged in a battle against the misinformation (Sun et al., 2022a) with informational tools. For instance, dashboards have been designed to track misinformation on social media and news-sharing platforms (e.g., COVID19MisInfo.org). Tencent, the largest social media platform operator in China runs a "Tencent Fact Check" (較真 in Chinese) program to debunk rumors about COVID-19. Also, WHO (2022) runs a "WHO myth busters" webpage to debunk inaccurate information related to COVID and a five-minute online game helping people learn strategies to resist misinformation and help stop the spread.

However, it was not clear how citizens from the four cities in our study take actions against the COVID-19 infodemic. Informed by the literature (Baek et al., 2019; Cheng & Luo, 2020) and building on our previous research (Lo et al., 2022; Wei et al., 2010), we examine in this chapter actions taken by respondents to counter the tsunami of COVID-19 misinformation.

DOI: 10.4324/9781003355984-10

Behavioral Responses to Perceived Impacts of Media Message

It is widely observed that biased perceptions of a public health risk will trigger behavioral responses (Wei et al., 2010). That is, when people believe others are more vulnerable to the influence of messages about public health than themselves, they will take actions according to that biased perception to address the perceived vulnerability of others (Gunther & Storey, 2003). Liu and Huang (2020) considered COVID-19 misinformation as a type of harmful message that would trigger people's biased perception of the general public as being more vulnerable than themselves, which then prompts them to take actions in reaction to that perception.

According to Sun et al. (2008), behavioral responses to biased perception can be grouped into three broad types: restrictive, corrective, and promotional. Though the taxonomies differ, restrictive action refers to support for restrictions or censorship of harmful content. Empirical evidence from studies on perceived influence of fake news, conspiracy theory, and misinformation related to the pandemic suggests a range of behavioral responses to control the harms of such messages. First, people will voice support for the government to regulate the messages (Baek et al., 2019). The American public was found to support governmental restrictions of misinformation during the COVID-19 pandemic (Cheng & Luo, 2020). Ho et al. (2022) reported that the presumed harms of fake science news on other scientists and the general public were positively associated with their attitude towards tackling fake science news, translating to support for legislative measures against fake science news.

Further, people may take actions to counterbalance the perceived imbalance or insufficiency of desirable information by sharing, advocating, or amplifying correct and positive messages. Sun et al. (2008) called it promotional action. In the context of the COVID-19 pandemic, the flood of misinformation has provoked institutions such as WHO and local and national health authorities to set up channels dedicated to promoting trusted COVID-19 information (Lo et al., 2022).

Finally, people may consider taking corrective actions. As Rojas (2010) suggested, this type of action is intended to correct what people perceive as "wrongs." The actions or activism varies. In combating misinformation related to COVID-19, several studies (Baek et al., 2019; Koo et al., 2021; Sun et al., 2022b) reported that people would take corrective action against misinformation when they believed the misinformation impacted the public.

Also, people's support for governmental restrictions of misinformation can further facilitate corrective action. Accordingly, we propose a type of civic action in combating COVID-19 misinformation. It includes assisting others by warning about suspicious messages on social media, sharing corrections of false information about the pandemic, and engaging in activism to fight misinformation for the sake of greater good.

Based on the above, we examined the respondents' three types of behavioral responses, including their support for government action to restrict COVID-19 misinformation, their own actions to counter the misinformation with correct scientific information as well as actions to help others to fight against the misinformation.

Operationally, our measures included the three types of behavioral responses with a total of 12 items adapted from the literature (Lo et al., 20022; Wei et al., 2010). To be specific, using a 5-point Likert scale, three statements measured support for governmental legislative action to restrict misinformation. They were: (1) COVID-19 misinformation should be regulated by the government; (2) COVID-19 misinformation should be censored by the government in accordance with the law; and (3) I support legislation to restrict the spread of COVID-19 misinformation ($M = 3.93$, $SD = .97$, $\alpha = .90$).

We then used a five-point scale ranging from 1 (never) to 5 (always) to measure the respondents' actions to promote correct and factually accurate information about the coronavirus. The three items were: (1) sharing correct information provided by World Health Organization; (2) sharing correct information provided by medical experts; and (3) sharing correct information that has been fact-checked ($M = 2.65$, $SD = .88$, $\alpha = .89$). To measure respondents' civic actions to combat misinformation, five items on a "1" (never) to "4" (often) scale were used: (1) alerting others about COVID-19 misinformation; (2) posting counter-arguments to misinformation concerning COVID-19; (3) posting corrections of COVID-19 misinformation; (4) sharing critical reviews of COVID-19 misinformation; (5) fact-checking the known misinformation about COVID-19 ($M = 2.45$, $SD = .80$, $\alpha = .89$).

Results of frequency analyses showed that support for government legislation to restrict misinformation related to COVID-19 was the most favored action among the 4,094 respondents in the four cities, followed by promotional and civic actions.

Findings

Patterns and Actions Taken to Combat Misinformation

To analyze behavioral responses, we conducted a series of *t*-tests or ANOVA to determine the difference in frequency of fighting-back actions taken by respondents with different demographic characteristics. Consistent with previous chapters, we first compared the respondents' differences in frequencies of engaging in actions to combat misinformation due to gender, age, education level, and city of residence (with low to high access to digital information). Results illuminated which respondents fought back against widespread misinformation on social media platforms, what type of actions they tended to take, and mechanisms (e.g., exposure and perception as triggers) underlying the process of taking different types of action.

In addition, respondents' fighting-back actions were compared based on their different levels of encountering with COVID-19 misinformation (low

level vs. high level of exposure and low-level vs. high-level of misinformation sharing), cognitive engagement with misinformation (low vs. high level
of elaboration), misinformation beliefs (low vs. high level of misbeliefs), and
knowledge about the pandemic (low vs. high level of knowledge). Measures
of elaboration, misbeliefs, and knowledge were provided in Chapter 8.

Gender Difference in Actions Against Misinformation

To compare the actions adopted by male and female respondents in the four
cities, an independent sample *t*-test was conducted. Results in Table 10.1 reveal
a significant gender difference in the overall frequency of actions to combat
misinformation ($t = 2.29$, $p < .05$). In general, male respondents ($M = 2.48$,
$SD = .81$) were more likely to take actions than female respondents ($M = 2.42$,
$SD = .80$) to restrict, correct, and debunk COVID-19 misinformation.

Among all types of actions to combat misinformation, the most frequent
action taken by both male and female respondents was fact-checking popular
yet debunked COVID-19 misinformation ($M = 2.75$; $M = 2.72$, respectively);
while the least frequent action taken by both male and female respondents
was sharing critical reviews of the COVID-19 misinformation ($M = 2.36$;
$M = 2.28$, respectively).

In terms of specific actions, some gender differences existed. Male
respondents ($M = 2.37$, $SD = 1.01$) reported a higher frequency of posting
counter-arguments against the COVID-19 misinformation than did female
respondents ($M = 2.29$, $SD = 1.00$), $t = 2.81$, $p < .01$. Also, male respondents

Table 10.1 Gender differences in actions to combat misinformation

	Male (n = 1,978)	Female (n = 2,116)	
	M (SD)	M (SD)	t value
1 Alerting others against the misinformation concerning COVID-19	2.53(.93)	2.50(.89)	1.09
2 Posting counter-argument of the misinformation concerning COVID-19	2.37(1.01)	2.29(1.00)	2.81**
3 Posting corrections of the misinformation concerning COVID-19	2.38(1.00)	2.33(.98)	1.69
4 Sharing critical reviews of the misinformation concerning COVID-19	2.36(.98)	2.28(.99)	2.75**
5 Checking the known misinformation concerning COVID-19	2.75(.94)	2.72(.93)	1.01
Combined index	2.48(.81)	2.42(.80)	2.29*

Note: The items were rated from 1 to 4, where 1 = never and 4 = often; M = mean, SD = standard
deviations; **$p < .01$, *$p < .05$.

(*M* = 2.36, *SD* = .98) also exhibited a higher frequency of sharing critical reviews of COVID-19 misinformation than did their female counterparts (*M* = 2.28, *SD* = .99). The difference was significant (*t* = 2.75, *p* < .01). However, there were no significant differences between male and female respondents in taking civic actions in terms of alerting others about COVID-19 misinformation (*t* = 1.09, *p* > .05), posting corrections (*t* = 1.69, *p* > .05) and fact-checking popular COVID-19 misinformation on social media (*t* = 1.01, *p* > .05).

Age Difference in Actions to Combat Misinformation

To discern whether the frequency of actions taken to combat misinformation differed by age groups, we split the age scale at the median to create two groups consisting of younger (*n* = 2,051) and older respondents (*n* = 2,042). Overall results (see Table 10.2) indicate that younger adults (*M* = 2.52, *SD* = .77) took actions more frequently than did older adults (*M* = 2.38, *SD* = .82), *t* = 5.94, *p* < .001.

The most frequent action by both age groups was fact-checking popular COVID-19 misinformation on social media outlets (*M* = 2.80; *M* = 2.67, respectively). The least frequent action taken by younger adults was sharing critical reviews of misinformation (*M* = 2.39); while the least frequent action taken by older adults was posting counter-arguments of the COVID-19 misinformation (*M* = 2.24).

As further illustrated in Table 10.2, compared to older adults, younger adults were more likely to take actions of all types, including alerting others of COVID-19 misinformation (*t* = 4.00, *p* < .001), posting counter-arguments (*t* = 5.68, *p* < .001), correcting the COVID-19 misinformation (*t* = 5.91,

Table 10.2 Differences in actions to combat misinformation between younger and older adults

	Younger adults (n = 2,051)	Older adults (n = 2,042)	
	M (SD)	M (SD)	t value
1 Alerting others against the misinformation concerning COVID-19	2.57(.89)	2.46(.93)	4.00***
2 Posting counter-argument of the misinformation concerning COVID-19	2.42(.99)	2.24(1.01)	5.68***
3 Posting corrections of the misinformation concerning COVID-19	2.44(.97)	2.26(1.00)	5.91***
4 Sharing critical reviews of the misinformation concerning COVID-19	2.39(.98)	2.25(.99)	4.38***
5 Checking the known misinformation concerning COVID-19	2.80(.91)	2.67(.96)	4.50***
Combined index	2.52(.77)	2.38(.82)	5.94***

Note: The items were rated from 1 to 4, where 1 = never and 4 = often; M = mean, SD = standard deviations; ***p < .001; the age entry has one missing value.

$p < .001$), sharing critical reviews of misinformation ($t = 4.38$, $p < .001$), and fact-checking the popularly spread COVID-19 misinformation online ($t = 4.50$, $p < .001$). These results suggest younger respondents across the four cities are more active in fighting back misinformation related to the pandemic.

Education and Actions to Combat Misinformation

To explore if education would make a difference in the frequency of taking actions to fight misinformation, we split the education scale at the median to generate two groups, respondents with a low level of education ($n = 1,528$) and respondents with a high level of education ($n = 2,566$). As results in Table 10.3 show, compared to respondents of a low level of education ($M = 2.34$, $SD = .81$), the overall frequency of taking actions to combat misinformation related to COVID-19 was significantly higher among respondents of a high level of education ($M = 2.52$, $SD = .78$). The difference was significant, $t = -6.56$, $p < .001$.

As detailed in Table 10.3, respondents with a high level of education were more frequently involved in all kinds of combating actions than those with a low level of education, including alerting others about the COVID-19 misinformation ($t = -4.42$, $p < .001$), posting counter-arguments ($t = -5.32$, $p < .001$), posting corrections ($t = -6.58$, $p < .001$), sharing critical reviews

Table 10.3 Differences in actions to combat misinformation between respondents of low and high level of education

	Low education (n = 1,528)	High education (n = 2,566)	
	M (SD)	*M (SD)*	*t value*
1 Alerting others against the misinformation concerning COVID-19	2.44(.93)	2.57(.90)	−4.42***
2 Posting counter-argument of the misinformation concerning COVID-19	2.22(1.01)	2.39(1.00)	−5.32***
3 Posting corrections of the misinformation concerning COVID-19	2.22(1.00)	2.43(.98)	−6.58***
4 Sharing critical reviews of the misinformation concerning COVID-19	2.23(.99)	2.37(.98)	−4.36***
5 Checking the known misinformation concerning COVID-19	2.61(.95)	2.81(.92)	−6.58***
Combined index	2.34(.81)	2.52(.78)	−6.56***

Note: The items were rated from 1 to 4, where 1 = never and 4 = often; M = mean, SD = standard deviations; ***p < .001.

($t = -4.36$, $p < .001$), and fact-checking the popularly diffused misinformation ($t = -6.58$, $p < .001$).

The least frequent actions taken by respondents with a low level of education were posting counter-arguments against COVID-19 misinformation ($M = 2.22$) and posting corrections ($M = 2.22$), while their most frequent action was fact-checking ($M = 2.61$). In comparison, the least frequent action taken by respondents with a high level of education was sharing critical reviews of COVID-19 misinformation ($M = 2.37$); while their most frequent action taken was fact-checking ($M = 2.81$).

Misinformation Exposure, Sharing, and Combating Actions

Next, to explore whether actions taken by respondents in the four cities to combat misinformation were tied to differences in exposure to COVID-19 misinformation as stimuli for behavioral responses, we divided the 4,094 respondents into two groups by splitting the misinformation exposure scale at the median. Accordingly, 1,858 respondents were categorized as low-exposure respondents and 2,236 as high-exposure respondents. Table 10.4 shows the results of independent-sample t-test, indicating a significant difference in the total actions taken to fight misinformation about COVID-19 between the low-exposure respondents and high-exposure respondents ($t = -21.05$, $p < .001$). High-exposure respondents ($M = 2.68$, $SD = .69$) reported more frequent overall actions than did low-exposure respondents ($M = 2.17$, $SD = .83$).

Table 10.4 Differences in actions to combat misinformation between respondents of low and high level of misinformation exposure

	Low exposure (n = 1,858)	High exposure (n = 2,236)	
	M (SD)	M (SD)	t value
1 Alerting others against the misinformation concerning COVID-19	2.29(.97)	2.71(.81)	−15.00***
2 Posting counter-argument of the misinformation concerning COVID-19	2.01(.98)	2.60(.95)	−19.50***
3 Posting corrections of the misinformation concerning COVID-19	2.05(.98)	2.61(.92)	−18.74***
4 Sharing critical reviews of the misinformation concerning COVID-19	2.02(.98)	2.57(.92)	−18.35***
5 Checking the known misinformation concerning COVID-19	2.50(1.00)	2.93(.84)	−14.75***
Combined index	2.17(.83)	2.68(.69)	−21.05***

Note: The items were rated from 1 to 4, where 1 = never and 4 = often; M = mean, SD = standard deviations; ***$p < .001$.

In terms of various types of fighting-back actions, high-exposure respondents took up the following counter-actions more frequently than did low-exposure respondents—alerting others to the COVID-19 misinformation ($t = -15.00$, $p < .001$), posting counter-arguments ($t = -19.50$, $p < .001$), posting corrections ($t = -18.74$, $p < .001$), sharing critical reviews ($t = -18.35$, $p < .001$), and fact-checking misinformation on social media ($t = -14.75$, $p < .001$).

The least frequent action taken by low-exposure respondents was posting counter-arguments ($M = 2.01$); while their most frequent action taken was fact-checking the debunked COVID-19 misinformation ($M = 2.50$). For respondents with a high level of misinformation exposure, the least frequently adopted behavior was sharing critical reviews of the COVID-19 misinformation ($M = 2.57$); while their most frequently adopted action was the same as the low-exposure respondents, i.e., fact-checking the COVID-19 misinformation ($M = 2.93$).

To further investigate whether respondents with different levels of sharing of misinformation exhibited similar patterns of taking various types of action, we distinguished respondents with a low-level ($n = 2,337$) and a high-level ($n = 1,757$) of misinformation sharing by splitting the misinformation sharing scale at the median. As *t*-test results in Table 10.5 show, the difference in overall frequency of actions to combat misinformation between the two groups was significant ($t = -27.87$, $p < .001$). Respondents with a high level of misinformation sharing ($M = 2.81$, $SD = .67$) engaged in combating actions more frequently than did those with a low level of misinformation sharing ($M = 2.18$, $SD = .78$).

In comparison to low-sharing respondents, high-sharing respondents more frequently alerted others to the COVID-19 misinformation ($t = -21.49$, $p < .001$), posted counter-arguments ($t = -26.37$, $p < .001$), posted corrections

Table 10.5 Differences in actions to combat misinformation between respondents of low and high level of misinformation sharing

	Low sharing (n = 2,337)	High sharing (n = 1,757)	
	M (SD)	M (SD)	t value
1 Alerting others against the misinformation concerning COVID-19	2.27(.92)	2.85(.78)	−21.49***
2 Posting counter-argument of the misinformation concerning COVID-19	2.00(.94)	2.77(.92)	−26.37***
3 Posting corrections of the misinformation concerning COVID-19	2.04(.94)	2.77(.89)	−25.16***
4 Sharing critical reviews of the misinformation concerning COVID-19	2.00(.94)	2.74(.88)	−25.84***
5 Checking the known misinformation concerning COVID-19	2.58(.99)	2.94(.82)	−12.67***
Combined index	2.18(.78)	2.81(.67)	−27.87***

Note: The items were rated from 1 to 4, where 1 = never and 4 = often; M = mean, SD = standard deviations; ***$p < .001$.

($t = -25.16$, $p < .001$), shared critical reviews ($t = -25.84$, $p < .001$), and fact-checked misinformation ($t = -12.67$, $p < .001$).

The least frequent actions by respondents with low-level misinformation sharing were posting counter-arguments ($M = 2.00$) and sharing critical reviews ($M = 2.00$), while their most frequently taken action was fact-checking ($M = 2.58$). In comparison, respondents with high-level misinformation sharing took this action the least frequently—sharing critical reviews of the misinformation ($M = 2.74$). As with low-sharing respondents, their most frequent action taken was fact-checking misinformation ($M = 2.94$). Taken together, these results highlight the role of exposure to and sharing of misinformation about COVID-19 in leading to respondents' combating actions.

Elaboration, Misbeliefs, Knowledge, and Combating Actions

To explore if the actions taken by respondents in the four cities to combat misinformation were related to differences in cognitive dimensions of processing COVID-19 misinformation that predict behavioral responses, we first classified the respondents by splitting the elaboration of misinformation scale at the median. Two groups were generated accordingly: low-elaboration ($n = 2,115$) and high-elaboration groups ($n = 1,979$). More t-tests were performed, results of which revealed a significant difference in the overall frequency of fighting-back actions between the two groups ($t = -23.23$, $p < .001$). As Table 10.6 shows, respondents with high-level elaboration ($M = 2.73$, $SD = .76$) were more frequently involved in actions to combat misinformation than those with low-level elaboration ($M = 2.19$, $SD = .74$). That is, cognitive efforts made to process the misinformation evoked actions to counter it.

Table 10.6 Differences in actions to combat misinformation between respondents of low and high level of misinformation elaboration

	Low elaboration ($n = 2,115$)	High elaboration ($n = 1,979$)	
	M (SD)	M (SD)	t value
1 Alerting others against the misinformation concerning COVID-19	2.26(.88)	2.79(.87)	−19.56***
2 Posting counter-argument of the misinformation concerning COVID-19	2.06(.92)	2.62(1.01)	−18.33***
3 Posting corrections of the misinformation concerning COVID-19	2.10(.93)	2.63(.98)	−17.61***
4 Sharing critical reviews of the misinformation concerning COVID-19	2.07(.93)	2.59(.98)	−17.50***
5 Checking the known misinformation concerning COVID-19	2.45(.92)	3.05(.86)	−21.56***
Combined index	2.19(.74)	2.73(.76)	−23.23***

Note: The items were rated from 1 to 4, where 1 = never and 4 = often; M = mean, SD = standard deviations; ***$p < .001$.

To be specific, low-elaboration respondents engaged significantly less often in the following actions than did those with high-elaboration—alerting others to the COVID-19 misinformation ($t = -19.56$, $p < .001$), posting counter-arguments against the misinformation ($t = -18.33$, $p < .001$), posting corrections ($t = -17.61$, $p < .001$), sharing critical reviews ($t = -17.50$, $p < .001$), and fact-checking ($t = -21.56$, $p < .001$).

Regarding the three types of actions to combat misinformation, the most frequent action taken by both low- and high-elaboration respondents was fact-checking ($M = 2.45$; $M = 3.05$, respectively). The least frequent action taken by low-elaboration respondents was posting counter-arguments against the misinformation ($M = 2.06$), while the least frequent action by high-elaboration respondents was sharing critical reviews ($M = 2.59$).

Similarly, to examine the variance of counter-actions adopted by respondents with different levels of misinformation beliefs, we divided respondents into low-level ($n = 2,066$) and high-level ($n = 2,028$) groups by splitting the misinformation belief scale at the median. As results presented in Table 10.7 indicate, there was a significant difference between the respondents with low vs. high level of misbeliefs in terms of their overall frequency of counter-actions ($t = -5.91$, $p < .001$).

Compared to respondents with a high level of misbeliefs, those with a low level reported significantly less frequent actions such as alerting others about the COVID-19 misinformation ($t = -3.30$, $p < .001$), posting counter-arguments ($t = -7.70$, $p < .001$), posting corrections ($t = -6.61$, $p < .001$), and sharing critical reviews ($t = -7.81$, $p < .001$). However, the difference in fact-checking between the two groups was not significant ($t = 1.38$, $p > .05$).

Table 10.7 Differences in actions to combat misinformation between respondents of low and high level of misinformation beliefs

	Low misbeliefs (n = 2,066)	High misbeliefs (n = 2,028)	
	M (SD)	M (SD)	t value
1 Alerting others against the misinformation concerning COVID-19	2.47(.95)	2.57(.86)	−3.30***
2 Posting counter-argument of the misinformation concerning COVID-19	2.21(1.01)	2.45(.99)	−7.70***
3 Posting corrections of the misinformation concerning COVID-19	2.25(1.01)	2.46(.95)	−6.61***
4 Sharing critical reviews of the misinformation concerning COVID-19	2.20(1.00)	2.44(.96)	−7.81***
5 Checking the known misinformation concerning COVID-19	2.76(.99)	2.72(.89)	1.38
Combined index	2.38(.83)	2.53(.76)	−5.91***

Note: The items were rated from 1 to 4, where 1 = never and 4 = often; M = mean, SD = standard deviations; ***$p < .001$.

With similar procedures, we further explored the differences in actions to combat misinformation between respondents with low and high levels of knowledge about the pandemic. The knowledge scale was split at the mean to classify the 4,094 respondents into two groups: respondents with low-level knowledge (n = 1,884) and respondents with high-level knowledge (n = 2,210). As illustrated in Table 10.8, the difference in the overall frequency of combating actions between respondents with low- and high-level knowledge (t = 4.27, p < .001) was significant. In general, respondents with low-level knowledge (M = 2.51, SD = .80) took fighting back actions more frequently than did those with high-level knowledge (M = 2.40, SD = .79).

Compared to respondents with high-level knowledge about COVID-19, respondents with low-level knowledge engaged in the following actions more frequently: alerting others to the COVID-19 misinformation (t = 2.33, p< .05), posting counter-arguments (t = 5.86, p < .001), posting corrections (t = 4.35, p < .001), and sharing critical reviews (t = 6.86, p < .001). However, it is worth noting that respondents with high-level knowledge were more frequently involved in fact-checking the popular misinformation on social media than were those with low-level knowledge (t = –2.08, p < .05).

Moreover, the least frequent action by respondents with high-level knowledge was sharing critical reviews of the COVID-19 misinformation (M = 2.22). Their most frequent action was fact-checking (M = 2.77). In comparison, the least frequent action by respondents with low-level knowledge was posting counter-arguments against the COVID-19 misinformation (M = 2.43), posting corrections (M = 2.43), and sharing critical reviews (M = 2.43); while their most frequent action was fact-checking (M = 2.70).

Table 10.8 Differences in actions to combat misinformation between respondents of low and high level of knowledge

	Low knowledge (n = 1,884)	High knowledge (n = 2,210)	
	M (SD)	M (SD)	t value
1 Alerting others against the misinformation concerning COVID-19	2.55(.90)	2.49(.92)	2.33*
2 Posting counter-argument of the misinformation concerning COVID-19	2.43(1.01)	2.24(1.00)	5.86***
3 Posting corrections of the misinformation concerning COVID-19	2.43(.99)	2.29(.98)	4.35***
4 Sharing critical reviews of the misinformation concerning COVID-19	2.43(.98)	2.22(.98)	6.86***
5 Checking the known misinformation concerning COVID-19	2.70(.94)	2.77(.93)	–2.08*
Combined index	2.51(.80)	2.40(.79)	4.27***

Note: The items were rated from 1 to 4, where 1 = never and 4 = often; M = mean, SD = standard deviations; ***p < .001.

City of Residence and Actions to Combat Misinformation

Did respondents in Beijing, Hong Kong, Taipei, and Singapore differ regarding actions to combat COVID-19 misinformation? To explore any city-based differences in behavioral responses, a series of ANOVA was conducted. Results presented in Table 10.9 indicate that respondents from the four cities differed in their overall actions to counter misinformation. The cross-city difference in the three types of fighting-back actions was significant, $F(3, 4090) = 124.24$, $p < .001$. Overall, Beijing respondents were the most active in taking counter actions ($M = 2.82$, $SD = .71$), followed by respondents from Singapore ($M = 2.45$, $SD = .78$), Taipei ($M = 2.30$, $SD = .83$), and Hong Kong ($M = 2.23$, $SD = .73$).

Table 10.9 further illustrates the significant differences among the respondents from the four cities in taking specific actions, including alerting others

Table 10.9 Differences in actions to combat misinformation among Beijing, Hong Kong, Taipei, and Singapore

	Beijing (n = 1,033)	Hong Kong (n = 1,017)	Taipei (n = 1,019)	Singapore (n = 1,025)	Total	F value
1 Alerting others against the misinformation concerning COVID-19	2.77(.86)	2.24(.86)	2.31(.93)	2.75(.85)	2.52(.91)	104.10***
2 Posting counter-argument of the misinformation concerning COVID-19	2.77(.95)	2.13(.95)	2.19(.98)	2.22(1.00)	2.33(1.01)	96.83***
3 Posting corrections of the misinformation concerning COVID-19	2.77(.94)	2.15(.90)	2.26(.98)	2.23(1.00)	2.35(.99)	90.76***
4 Sharing critical reviews of the misinformation concerning COVID-19	2.77(.93)	2.06(.90)	2.11(.95)	2.34(1.00)	2.32(.99)	120.58***
5 Checking the known misinformation concerning COVID-19	3.04(.87)	2.55(.90)	2.63(.98)	2.73(.93)	2.74(.94)	55.66***
Combined index	2.82(.71)	2.23(.73)	2.30(.83)	2.45(.78)	2.45(.80)	124.24***

Note: The items were rated from 1 to 4, where 1 = never and 4 = often; ***$p < .001$.

about the COVID-19 misinformation [$F(3, 4090) = 104.10, p < .001$], posting counter-arguments [$F(3, 4090) = 96.83, p < .001$], posting corrections [$F(3, 4090) = 90.76, p < .001$], sharing critical reviews [$F(3, 4090) = 120.58, p < .001$], and fact-checking [$F(3, 4090) = 55.66, p < .001$].

Across the four cities, the most frequent action of Beijing respondents was fact-checking the COVID-19 misinformation ($M = 3.04, SD = .87$), and other types of actions such as sharing critical reviews. Hong Kong respondents' most frequent counter-action was fact-checking the misinformation ($M = 2.55, SD = .90$) whereas their least frequent counter-action was sharing critical reviews ($M = 2.06, SD = .90$). Taipei respondents engaged in fact-checking the misinformation ($M = 2.63, SD = .98$) the most frequently and posted counter-arguments against the misinformation ($M = 2.11, SD = .95$) the least frequently.

The behavioral responses among the Singaporean respondents were unique. Unlike respondents in the other three cities, the most frequent counter-action undertaken by Singapore respondents was alerting others to COVID-19 misinformation ($M = 2.75, SD = .85$) whereas their least frequent combating action was posting counter-arguments ($M = 2.22, SD = 1.00$). These results suggest encountering misinformation about COVID-19 stimulates behavioral responses to misinformation. Respondents in Beijing who were exposed the most to such information took actions to fight back the most often.

Predicting Actions to Combat Misinformation

Finally, to understand why respondents fight back against misinformation, we performed multivariate analyses to identify the most significant predictors (e.g., misinformation exposure, sharing, elaboration, misbeliefs, and knowledge) of the three types of actions (i.e., support for restrictive action by the government, promotional and civic actions). Three hierarchical regression analyses were conducted, treating support for government action to restrict misinformation, promotional action, and civic action, respectively, as the dependent variables. For the predictors, demographic variables, including age, gender, education, and city of residence were entered in Block 1 as control variables, followed by misinformation exposure in Block 2 and misinformation sharing in Block 3. Elaboration was entered in Block 4, misinformation beliefs were entered in Block 5, and knowledge was entered in Block 6.

As results in Table 10.10 show, city of residence was a significant predictor of the three types of actions to combat misinformation. Respondents who were living in Beijing more frequently engaged in overall counter-actions.

More importantly, exposure to misinformation was a strong and significant predictor of how frequently people were involved in all three types of action against misinformation ($\beta = .10, p < .001$ for support of restrictive action by the government; $\beta = .20, p < .001$ for promotional actions; and $\beta = .20, p < .001$ for civic actions). Misinformation sharing was significantly related to promotional actions ($\beta = .22, p < .001$) and civic actions ($\beta = .27, p < .001$), but not support for government actions. Elaboration turned out to be a consistent predictor of all three types of actions (β = .28, p < .001 for support of government action to restrict misinformation; β = .25, p < .001 for promotional actions; β = .27, p < .001 for civic actions). In addition, misbeliefs were significantly related only to support of government action to restrict misinformation (β = –.17, p < .001) and civic actions (β = .04, p < .05). Respondents who formed more misbeliefs about COVID-19 corrected misinformation more often but were not supportive of restrictive government actions.

In terms of variance, the significant predictors explained well the three types of combating actions taken by respondents (35.1% for civic actions, 26.5% for promotional actions, and 16.3% for support of government action). These results suggest that exposure to, sharing of, and elaboration about misinformation explain how often respondents in the four cities took actions to combat misinformation during the pandemic. That is, the greater the exposure to, sharing of, and elaboration about misinformation, the more often the respondents engaged in actions against misinformation on social media outlets.

Table 10.10 Hierarchical regression analyses predicting actions to combat misinformation

Predictors	Support for restrictions of misinformation	Taking Promotional actions	Taking Civic Actions
Block 1: Demographics			
Age	.08***	.04**	–.02
Gender (Male = 1)	–.04**	–.01	.02
Education	–.01	.01	.05**
City (1 = Beijing)	.19***	.15***	.12***
Adjusted R^2	6.4%	7.8%	8.8%
Block 2: Misinformation exposure			
Misinformation exposure	.10***	.20***	.20***
Incremental adjusted R^2	0.2%	8.1%	12.2%
Block 3: Misinformation sharing			
Misinformation sharing	–.01	.22***	.27***
Incremental adjusted R^2	0.0%	4.7%	7.6%
Block 4: Elaboration			
Elaboration	.28***	.25***	.27***
Incremental adjusted R^2	8.0%	5.9%	6.4%
Block 5: Misinformation beliefs			
Misinformation beliefs	–.17***	–.03	.04*
Incremental adjusted R^2	1.8%	0.0%	0.1%
Block 6: Knowledge			
Knowledge	–.01	.03	.00
Incremental adjusted R^2	0.0%	0.0%	0.0%
Total adjusted R^2	16.3%	26.5%	35.1%

Note: Beijing was coded as 1 and other cities were coded as 0; N = 4,093; ***p < .001; **p < .01; The age entry has one missing value

Summary of Key Findings

This chapter's presentation of quantitative findings regarding the behavioral responses to misinformation revealed patterns of taking different types of actions to combat the misinformation on social media:

- Across the board, support for the government action to restrict misinformation related to COVID-19 by legislation was the most favored action against misinformation among the 4,094 respondents in the four cities, followed by promotional and civic actions taken by citizens (i.e., fact-checking the COVID-19 misinformation).
- Male respondents took fighting-back actions more frequently than did female respondents, especially with regard to posting counter-arguments and sharing critical reviews of misinformation.
- In general, younger respondents more frequently engaged in all three types of actions to combat misinformation than did older respondents. Also, respondents with a high level of education engaged in three kinds of combating actions more frequently than did those with a low level of education.
- As consumers and disseminators of misinformation, compared to low exposure and sharing respondents, respondents with high exposure and more frequent sharing took all three types of fighting-back actions more frequently. Moreover, the frequency of actions to fight against misinformation was higher among respondents who elaborated more about misinformation and those with high-level of misinformation beliefs.
- It is noteworthy that respondents with low-level knowledge about COVID-19 generally engaged in counter-actions more frequently than did those with high-level knowledge. They also differed in types of actions.
- Among the four cities, Beijing respondents were the most active in combating actions most frequently, followed by respondents from Singapore, Taipei, and Hong Kong.
- Regression results showed significant predictors of the frequency of taking actions against misinformation: exposure, sharing, misbeliefs, and elaboration. They explained the three types of combating actions with varying degrees of success (35.1% for civic actions, 26.5% for promotional actions, and 16.5% for support of government action).

Qualitative Findings

The personal accounts of focus group participants provided nuanced insights into the reasoning behind taking or not taking action to counter misinformation on social media. Their accounts are revealing and insightful.

Let it go: Reasons for Non-Action

Mr. Wu, a 36-year-old male participant from Beijing, said that everyone was caught unprepared for the outbreaks. Beijing residents panicked and lined up to stock up on food and traditional Chinese herbal medicines during the initial outbreaks. "When I saw the public panic," he recounted, "I was worried too. But I said to friends around me: Stay calm. If residents of Beijing face a food shortage, what about the rest of the country?" He believed that people of wisdom would stop the rumors and misinformation.

Unlike him, another 54-year-old male education institution manager from Beijing Mr. He said he decided to do nothing about the misinformation spread on social media. His reasoning: "In the information age, transparency takes care of itself. Falsehood will lose to credible information. I do not counter it with any action. Rather, I just laugh it out. I simply take those ridiculous misinformation messages as a joke."

A younger male participant in Singapore Jack also told a story about sharing COVID-19 misinformation as a joke. According to his account,

> A YouTube video mocking Trump, saying that drinking bleach can cure COVID. Uh, I think I did share it with my family. We just had a lot [of fun] about it. But I yeah, we just think like how can anybody take him seriously after this?

Olivia, a female student in Hong Kong, shared a similar story. She said when facial masks were in short supply in the territory of nearly 8 million residents, a posting on Facebook asserted that steamed facial masks could be reused. She said, "We shared this piece of misinformation message among friends as a joke. It simply does not make sense because steaming does not cleanse the virus."

The third male participant from Beijing Mr. Guo, who is 43 years old and works in IT, added another perspective—the importance of knowledge. He explained,

> Living with COVID for two years has taught me a great deal, including encountering a bunch of false or misleading messages about the disease. These messages cannot pass the test of common sense. If you bother to fact check or debunk the false information (on social media), people might say, we already know it. Why don't you?

Theodore, a 26-year-old male sales rep working in Singapore, echoed him. He cited several examples of misinformation to kill the virus such as drinking bleach, hanging a necklace or pendant, and putting a mosquito patch on the chest. He summed it up by saying, "Those are the things you don't really need to fact-check. It's common sense, right?" A male participant in Taipei did the same—simply ignoring the false information about COVID-19 spread on social media. Mr. Chang, the 33-year-old male flight attendant said,

> My dad viewed tons of videos on mainland China's social media site and he would tell me some of those false videos on how to prevent infections with diet and herbs. I did not believe any of that stuff. I didn't bother to fact check, either. I would rather believe they were false.

Another 37-year-old female fashion designer in Singapore, Abigail, explained her reaction to suspicious news about COVID-19 on WhatsApp. She said,

> I realize all this news being shared is usually from the elderly, uncles or aunties, they're usually the first few who share all this information. Let's say the person is close to me like my parents, my family, I can ask them, don't share to so many people in case it's fake. Yeah, I will advise them but if it's just my friends, I would usually just ignore this. It's up to you whether you want to share.

Ms. Hsieh, a 39-year-old female in Taipei had the same idea, "I would totally ignore the misleading and false posts," she said.

> Even when I was tested positive, my mom kept forwarding me information about long-term harms of infection like damaged brain, blah blah. I asked her to stop sending me those messages without evidence. I did not bother to fact check at all because as someone being tested positive, I knew my brain was just fine.

Another female participant Sofia, a 50-year-old sales manager in Singapore, simply chose to tune out from the noise on Facebook. She said, "I block all those [notifications] so I don't get them." Abigail, the female also from Singapore, said something similar, emphasizing one's common sense. "I actually welcome all this news that I receive on those messages on WhatsApp," she explained.

> I like to receive and I like to listen or read them and I will decide whether to believe it or not. And I usually won't ask them to stop sending, stop circulating or tell them it's fake news because once they share, they somehow believe it. So, I don't think I'm in a position to like, discredit them from all this information they send because they care. So, I usually won't stop them unless they're my parents or I tell them, "Yeah, fake one". Don't listen. OK. Other than that, I will just ignore. Just read them. Uh, decide yourself whether you want to listen or not.

Striking Back

A male student in Taipei Mr. Hung indicated that he often took action against COVID-19 misinformation. "A couple of my close friends and family members, mostly the elderly, had the habit of sharing with me false posts about COVID almost every day," he recalled.

> I was clueless whether those posts were true or not. I then fact checked them online. I sent the results to my friends and family with screen shots of the results to embarrasses them. Soon, they cut down sharing

with me those half-truths. I would show them that the messages were false right on their face.

Amelia, a 39-year-old housewife in Hong Kong, said she fact-checked specific misinformation about infected restaurants and reported the fact-checked information to her family members for attention. She explained,

> I am so tired and sick of so many misleading updates on closures of restaurants where people were tested positive, I would go to the government site to fact check them. Then, I let my family know about those false messages.

Mr. Chou aged 55 from Taipei, was knowledgeable about the pandemic and often fact-checked misleading messages or half-truths. He said, "I would discuss those posts with friends, and send a warning about those posts to everyone to watch out for the trickery."

On the other hand, actions taken by average citizens may have unexpected consequences. According to Mr. Ma from Beijing, a friend of his in his 60s worked in a hospital in Beijing. The hospital worker, who was near his retirement, mentioned in his personal posting on WeChat that vaccines can expire. When expired, a shot would be useless. He was taken into custody by the authorities for the post to his friends.

Conclusion and Insights

In sum, analysis of the quantitative data shed light on the question of who would take actions to fight back against widely diffused COVID-19 misinformation on social media. In addition to key demographics, we identified several key variables such as exposure, sharing, elaboration, and misbeliefs that played very important roles in explaining respondents' actions to combat misinformation. These factors function as the stimulus and cognitive mechanisms that evoked actions against misinformation. For instance, respondents who thought more about the consequences of misinformation (high level of elaboration) took actions more frequently to combat misinformation. That is, cognitive efforts to process the misinformation evoked action to counter falsehoods. These results validated our analytical framework of stimulus-orientation-response proposed in Chapter 1.

The insights to be drawn from these key findings are that flattening the curve of infodemic during a pandemic requires the actions of all sectors of a society, both the government and citizens. Our findings indicate that citizens' action is particularly critical in combating the waves of false, misleading, and factually incorrect information on leading social media platforms. Further, citizens with better educations who take efforts to process the misinformation they encounter on social media are most active in fighting back. Also, those with high-level knowledge about the pandemic tend to do more fact-checking of misinformation than those with low-level knowledge. Thus, government and public health officials should mobilize better-educated citizens to contest misinformation. At the same time, public health websites and social media need to provide detailed factual information to arm citizens with the needed knowledge to identify and debunk half-truths during a pandemic.

References

Baek, Y., Kang, H., & Kim, S. (2019). Fake news should be regulated because it influences both "others" and "me": How and why the influence of presumed influence model should be extended. *Mass Communication & Society, 22*(3), 301–323. https://doi.org/10.1080/15205436.2018.1562076

Cheng, Y., & Luo, Y. (2020). The presumed influence of digital misinformation: Examining US public's support for governmental restrictions versus corrective action in the COVID-19 pandemic. *Online Information Review, 45*(4), 834–852. https://doi.org/10.1108/OIR-08-2020-0386

Gunther, A., & Storey, J. (2003). The influence of presumed influence. *Journal of Communication, 53*(2), 199–215. https://doi.org/10.1111/j.1460-2466.2003.tb02586.x

Ho, S. S., Goh, T. J., & Leung, Y. W. (2022). Let's nab fake science news: Predicting scientists' support for interventions using the influence of presumed media influence model. *Journalism, 23*(4), 910–928. https://doi.org/10.1177/1464884920937488

Koo, A., Su, M., Lee, S., Ahn, S., & Rojas, H. (2021). What motivates people to correct misinformation? Examining the effects of third-person perceptions and perceived Norms. *Journal of Broadcasting & Electronic Media, 65*(1), 111–134. https://doi.org/10.1080/08838151.2021.1903896

Liu, P., & Huang, L. (2020). Digital disinformation about COVID-19 and the third-person effect: Examining the channel differences and negative emotional outcomes. *Cyberpsychology, Behavior, and Social Networking, 23*(11), 789–793. https://doi.org/10.1089/cyber.2020.0363

Lo, V., Wei, R., Lu, M., Zhang, X., & Qiu, J. L. (2022, May). *A comparative study of the impact of digital media environments, information processing and presumed influence on behavioral responses to COVID-19 misinformation in four Asian cities* [Paper presentation]. International Communication Association Annual Conference 2022, Paris, France.

Rojas, H. (2010). "Corrective" action in the public sphere: How perceptions of media and media effects shape political behaviors. *International Journal of Public Opinion Research, 22*(3), 343–363. https://doi.org/10.1093/ijpor/edq018

Sun, Y., Chia, S. C., Lu, F., & Oktavianus, J. (2022a). The battle is on: Factors that motivate people to combat anti-vaccine misinformation. *Health Communication, 37*(3), 327–336. https://doi.org/10.1080/10410236.2020.1838108

Sun, Y., Oktavianus, J., Wang, S., & Lu, F. (2022b, 2022/09/19). The role of influence of presumed influence and anticipated guilt in evoking social correction of COVID-19 misinformation. *Health Communication, 37*(11), 1368–1377. https://doi.org/10.1080/10410236.2021.1888452

Sun, Y., Shen, L., & Pan, Z. (2008). On the behavioral component of the third-person effect. *Communication Research, 35*(2), 257–278. https://doi.org/10.1177/009365020731316

Wei, R., Lo, V., & Lu, H. (2010). The third-person effect of tainted food product recall news: Examining the role of credibility, attention, and elaboration for college students in Taiwan. *Journalism & Mass Communication Quarterly, 87*(3–4), 598–614. https://doi.org/10.1177/107769901008700310

WHO. (2022). *Coronavirus disease (COVID-19) advice for the public: Myth-busters*. World Health Organization. https://www.who.int/emergencies/diseases/novel-coronavirus-2019/advice-for-public/myth-busters

11 Modeling the Dynamic Process and Adverse Effects of Misinformation

Ven-Hwei Lo and Ran Wei

Introduction

Building on the bivariate and multivariate analyses discussed in Chapters 4–10, this chapter further explores the process and effects of misinformation about COVID with a causal modeling approach. Structural modeling (Bollen, 1989) is superior to regression-based predictive modeling in providing a holistic view of the causal chains from societal factors as antecedents to encountering misinformation. These factors account for a range of affective, cognitive, attitudinal, and behavioral effects (Bagozzi & Yi, 2012). For example, causal mechanism (technically called "causal structure") can be clarified from a range of significant predictors to reveal the dynamics in cause and effect relationships. At the same time, the direct and indirect effects of antecedents on predictors and outcome variables can be clarified in inferring causal conclusions.

In addition to the structural equation modeling (SEM) approach, we used a statistical technique called mediation analysis (Hayes, 2017) to assess the mediating effects of identified causal mechanisms. One such mechanism includes moderators, defined as factors that influence the level, direction, or presence of a relationship between variables. Moderators show for whom, when, or under what circumstances a relationship between an independent and outcome variable holds. Another mechanism includes mediators, defined as intermediate variables that explain how an independent variable influences an outcome variable. Because mediation assumes both causality and a temporal ordering (Gunzler et al., 2013), additional insights about causal structure can be drawn.

Technically, in running process to examine mediation and moderation, a statistical procedure called boot-strapping is typically used. Boot-strapping refers to resampling a single dataset to create many simulated samples with much larger sample size such as 5,000 at 95% or 99% confidence intervals (Kulesa et al., 2015).

DOI: 10.4324/9781003355984-11

Findings

Sharing Behavior of Misinformation

To build a causal model on exposure to and sharing of misinformation about COVID-19, we used the results of the regression analyses of the online survey data as the basis (refer to Table 4.12 in Chapter 4). Our theoretical model is presented in Figure 11.1, which shows that information accessibility will affect exposure to COVID-19 misinformation and perceived interest of others in COVID-19 information, which will in turn affect misinformation-sharing behaviors. The model will address our RQ1: How does digital information accessibility in society affect the sharing of COVID misinformation through exposure to misinformation and perceived interests of others, which motivate citizens' misinformation-sharing behavior?

To test the proposed model, we implemented SEM using *Amos* 27. The results of the analyses show that although the chi-square for the model was significant, $X^2 = 1,031.65$, $df = 69$, $p < .001$ (X^2/df ratio = 14.95), the comparative fit index (CFI) value of .99, the normal fit index (NFI) value of .99, and the Tucker–Lewis index (TLI) value of .97, together with the root mean square error of approximation (RMSEA) value of .06 indicate that the model fit was very good. The model explained 4.0% of the variance in exposure to COVID-19 misinformation, 10.6% of the variance in perceived interest of others, 34.5% in misinformation sharing, and 39.7% in number of people shared.

In terms of strengths of the linkages between the exogenous variables and the endogenous variables, as further shown in Figure 11.1, the structural equation model shows that information accessibility had a significant impact on exposure to COVID-19 misinformation ($\beta = -.22$, $p < .001$), and perceived

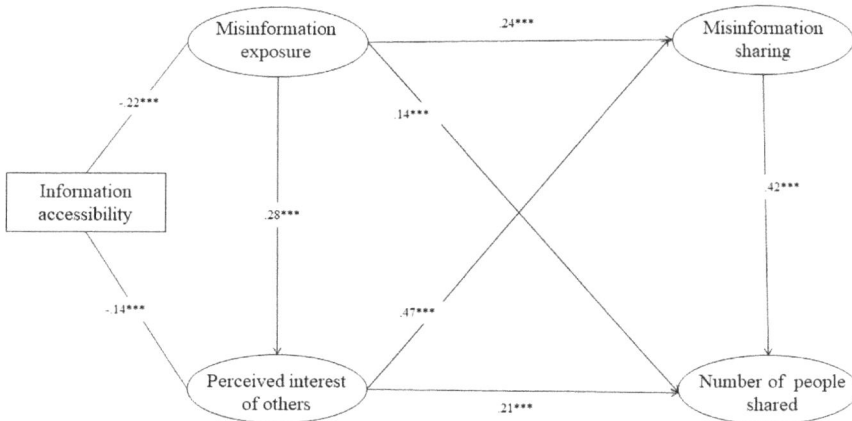

Figure 11.1 Structural equation model of predictors of misinformation sharing

interest of others (β = –.14, p < .001). Exposure to COVID-19 misinformation had a significant effect on perceived interest of others (β = .28, p < .001), misinformation sharing (β = .24, p < .001), and number of people shared (β = .14, p < .001). Further, perceived interest of others had a significant effect on misinformation sharing (β = .47, p < .001), and number of people shared (β = .21, p < .001). Finally, misinformation sharing was significantly associated with number of people shared (β = .42 p < .001).

Taken together, the structural equation model results indicate that information accessibility tends to have a negative and direct impact on exposure to COVID-19 misinformation and perceived interest of others and have a negative and indirect influence on misinformation-sharing behaviors. What these results mean is that exposure to COVID-19 misinformation and perceived interest of others are significant mediators of the relationship between information accessibility and misinformation-sharing behaviors.

To further assess the mediating effects of exposure to COVID-19 misinformation and perceived interest of others in the relationships between information accessibility and misinformation-sharing behaviors, we adopted a procedure developed by Sobel (1982) that provides a direct test of an indirect effect. The two mediators in our theoretical model are exposure to COVID-19 misinformation and perceived interest of others. The results of the Sobel test indicate that exposure to COVID-19 misinformation significantly mediated the relationships between information accessibility and misinformation sharing (z = –12.23, p < .001) and between information accessibility and number of people shared (z = –12.34, p < .001). The results of the Sobel test also indicate that perceived interest of others significantly mediated the relationships between information accessibility and misinformation sharing (z = –12.35, p < .001) and between information accessibility and number of people shared (z = –12.12, p < .001).

To ascertain the mediating effects of exposure to COVID-19 misinformation and perceived interest of others in the relationship between information accessibility and misinformation-sharing behaviors, an additional bootstrapping procedure was conducted using the SPSS version of PROCESS macro model 4 (Hayes, 2017). The bootstrap method demonstrates that the mediating effects we reported with the Sobel test were accurate and appropriate. Specifically, the bootstrapping procedure was used with 5,000 bootstrap samples and 95% bias-corrected bootstrap-confidence intervals.

The results showed that exposure to COVID-19 misinformation was a significant mediator of the relationship between information accessibility and misinformation sharing (β = –.06, SE = .01, 95% CI = [–.073, –.049]). Moreover, the indirect effect of information accessibility on number of people shared through exposure to COVID-19 misinformation was also significant (β = –.12, SE = .01, 95% CI = [–.141, –.102]). Additionally, perceived interest of others significantly mediated the effect of information accessibility on misinformation sharing (β = –.24, SE = .03, 95% CI = [–.294, –.194]) and number of people shared (β = –.36, SE = .03, 95% CI = [–.423, –.301]).

These findings answered our RQ1: the increased exposure to COVID-19 misinformation and perceived interest of others caused by information accessibility led to stronger misinformation-sharing behaviors.

Consequences of Sharing of Misinformation

Next, to explore how information accessibility, exposure to misinformation, and sharing of misinformation affected people's beliefs, attitudes, and knowledge about the pandemic, we developed another theoretical model. The model is depicted in Figure 11.2. We specified the model as starting with information accessibility, exposure to COVID-19 misinformation, misinformation sharing, misinformation beliefs, anti-vaccine attitudes, and knowledge about COVID-19. We estimated that information accessibility would directly predict exposure to misinformation and misinformation sharing, which in turn would predict misinformation beliefs, anti-vaccine attitudes, and knowledge about COVID-19. Results of the model would thus address our RQ2: How does digital information accessibility in society directly affect respondents' encounters with COVID misinformation and indirectly impact their cognitive and attitudinal responses?

To test the model, we took the SEM approach. Results showed that the overall chi-square value for the model was significant, (χ^2 = 2,049.76, df =89, χ^2/df = 23.03, p < .001). The baseline comparisons fit indices indicated that the model fit was acceptable with the CFI value of .95, the NFI value of .94, the TLI of .93, and the RMSEA value of .07. The model explained 4.2% of the variance in exposure to misinformation, 15.7% variance in misinformation sharing, 9.4% variance in anti-vaccine attitudes, 41.7% in misinformation beliefs, and 3.8% in knowledge about COVID-19.

As Figure 11.2 shows, the structural equation model indicated that information accessibility had a direct but negative effect on exposure to COVID-19 misinformation (β = −.21, p < .001) and misinformation sharing (β = −.07, p < .001). Exposure to COVID-19 misinformation had a significant positive effect on misinformation sharing (β = .37, p < .001), misinformation beliefs (β = .57, p < .001), anti-vaccine attitudes (β = .26, p < .001), and knowledge about COVID-19 (β = −.08, p < .001). Misinformation sharing also had a significant effect on misinformation beliefs (β = .15, p < .001), anti-vaccine attitudes (β = .09, p < .001), and knowledge about COVID-19 (β = −.15, p < .001).

We next conducted mediation analyses to test the direct and indirect effects of information accessibility on misinformation beliefs, anti-vaccine attitudes, and knowledge about COVID-19. We were interested in exploring *whether* and *how* exposure to misinformation and misinformation sharing would mediate the impact of information accessibility on misinformation beliefs, anti-vaccine attitudes, and knowledge about COVID-19.

A total of six Sobel tests were conducted. Results show that exposure to COVID misinformation was a significant mediator in the relationship between information accessibility and misinformation beliefs (z = −13.24,

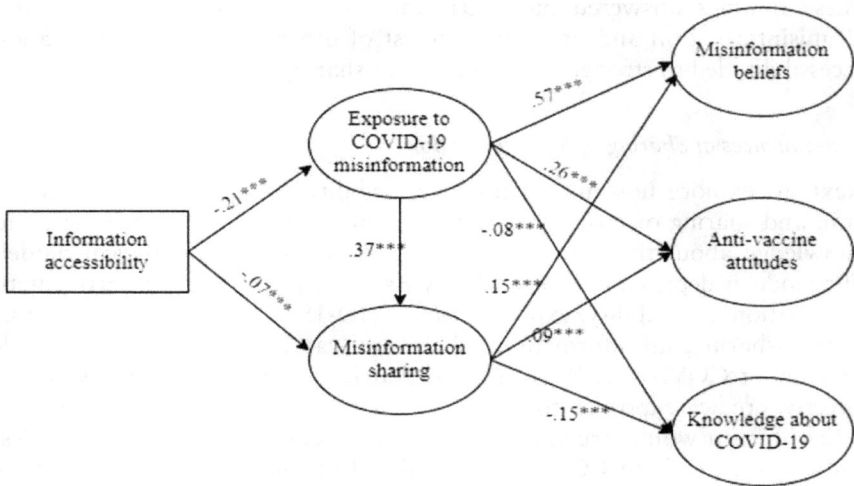

Figure 11.2 Structural equation model of predictors of cognitive and attitudinal outcomes

$p < .001$), anti-vaccine attitudes ($z = -11.11$, $p < .001$), and knowledge about COVID-19 ($z = 6.66$, $p < .001$). Similarly, misinformation sharing was a significant mediator in the relationship between information accessibility and misinformation beliefs ($z = -8.92$, $p < .001$), anti-vaccine attitudes ($z = -7.45$, $p < .001$), and knowledge about COVID-19 ($z = 7.48$, $p < .001$). These results indicate that exposure to misinformation and misinformation sharing were statistically significant mediators in the relationship between information accessibility and the three cognitive and attitudinal outcomes.

An additional bootstrap test also demonstrated that exposure to COVID-19 misinformation and misinformation sharing were significant mediators in the relationships between information accessibility and misinformation misbeliefs, anti-vaccine attitudes, and knowledge about COVID. The results showed that exposure to COVID-19 misinformation was a significant mediator of the relationship between information accessibility and misinformation belief ($\beta = -.12$, $SE = .01$, 95% CI = $[-.142, -.102]$). Moreover, the indirect effect of information accessibility on anti-vaccine attitudes ($\beta = -.08$, $SE = .01$, 95% CI = $[-.099, -.068]$) and knowledge about COVID-19 ($\beta = -.02$, $SE = .01$, 95% CI = $[.010, .037]$) through exposure to COVID-19 misinformation were also significant. In addition, misinformation sharing significantly mediated the effect of information accessibility on misinformation beliefs ($\beta = -.03$, $SE = .00$, 95% CI = $[-.036, -.021]$), anti-vaccine attitudes ($\beta = -.03$, $SE = .00$, 95% CI = $[-.033, -.017]$), and knowledge about COVID-19 ($\beta = .04$, $SE = .01$, 95% CI = $[.032, .059]$).

Effects of Perceived Influence of Misinformation

Next, to explore the presumed influence of COVID-19 misinformation on respondents' behavioral responses, we developed an integrated model based on the influence of presumed influence model (Gunther & Storey, 2003) and the information-processing theory (McGuire, 1978). This third model was advantageous for articulating the theoretical linkages among digital information accessibility, exposure, and key information-processing variables, presumed influence of misinformation, negative emotions, and behavioral responses. We intended to use it to address our third RQ3: how does digital information accessibility as an exogenous variable affect respondents' exposure to COVID-19 misinformation that impacts their perceived effects of the misinformation, which trigger behavioral responses to contain the misinformation?

As Figure 11.3 illustrates, the model showed that digital information accessibility affected levels of exposure to misinformation, which led to elaboration of misinformation, which led to presumed influence of misinformation, which elicited negative emotions, which in turn prompted respondents to take restrictive, promotional, and correction actions.

To test the model, another structural equation model was employed. Results of the SEM showed that the model fit was adequate (χ^2 = 3,297.04, df = 326, χ^2/df = 10.11, $p < .001$; CFI = .96, TLI = .96, NFI = .95, RMSEA = .047). The model explained 5.1% of the variance in exposure to misinformation, 6.7% in elaboration of misinformation, 26.7% in presumed influence of misinformation, 51% in negative emotions, 22.9% in support for government restrictions of misinformation, 26.9% in promotional behavior, and 29.4% in action to counter misinformation.

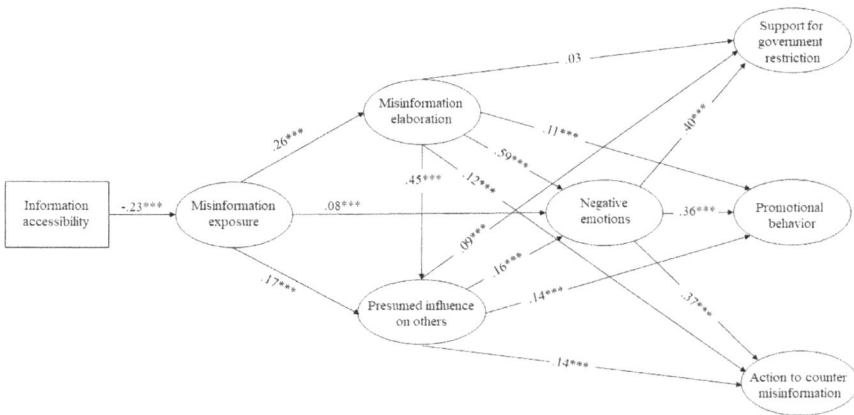

Figure 11.3 Structural equation model of predictors of support for behavioral responses to counter misinformation

In terms of strengths of the linkage among the eight variables in the model, information accessibility had a significant and direct impact on exposure to misinformation ($\beta = -.23$, $p < .001$). As Figure 11.3 shows, exposure to misinformation had a significant and direct impact on misinformation elaboration ($\beta = .26$, $p < .001$), presumed influence of misinformation on others ($\beta = .17$, $p < .001$), and negative emotions ($\beta = .08$, $p < .001$). Misinformation elaboration had a significant and direct effect on presumed influence of misinformation on others ($\beta = .45$, $p < .001$), negative emotions ($\beta = .59$, $p < .001$), promotional behavior ($\beta = .11$, $p < .001$), and action to counter misinformation ($\beta = .12$, $p < .001$). Presumed influence of misinformation on others was significantly related to negative emotions ($\beta = .16$, $p < .001$), support for government restriction ($\beta = .09$, $p < .001$), promotional behavior ($\beta = .14$, $p < .001$), and action to counter misinformation ($\beta = .14$, $p < .001$). Finally, negative emotions had a significant and positive effect on support for government restriction ($\beta = .40$, $p < .001$), promotional behavior ($\beta = .36$, $p < .001$), and action to counter misinformation ($\beta = .37$, $p < .001$).

These SEM results revealed how digital information accessibility affected exposure to COVID misinformation and elaboration of such misinformation, which led to presumed influence, and several behavioral responses to contain COVID misinformation through negative emotions. The linkages among these variables in our integrated model suggest elaboration and presumed influence as critical cognitive mechanisms in understanding the effects of exposure to misinformation on behavioral responses to misinformation.

Furthermore, to assess the mediating effects of negative emotions in mitigating the effects of presumed influence of misinformation on others on the three health behaviors, we adopted the Sobel test. The results indicate that negative emotions significantly mediated the relationships between presumed influence of misinformation on others and support for government restriction of misinformation ($z = 20.50$, $p < .001$), between presumed influence of misinformation on others and promotional behavior ($z = 20.28$, $p < .001$) and between presumed influence of misinformation on others and action to counter misinformation ($z = 21.51$, $p < .001$).

To assess the mediating effects of negative emotions mitigating the effects of presumed influence of misinformation on support for government restriction, promotional behavior, and action to counter misinformation, we also adopted the bootstrapping procedure developed by Hayes (2013). Results of the bootstrapping procedure show that presumed influence of misinformation was indirectly associated with support for government restriction ($\beta = .18$, $SE = .02$, 95% CI = [.153, .185), promotional behavior ($\beta = .16$, $SE = .02$, 95% CI = [.137, .203]), and actions to counter misinformation ($\beta = .15$, $SE = .01$, 95% CI = [.136, .172]) via negative emotions. Thus, the bootstrapping procedure confirmed that negative emotions were a significant mediator in the relationships between presumed influence and support for government restriction, promotional behavior, and action to counter misinformation.

Government Trust as a Moderator of Action to Restrict Misinformation

Finally, we raised RQ4 to explore whether and how trust in government moderates the relationship between misinformation exposure and presumed influence of misinformation and the relationship between presumed influence of misinformation and support for government restriction of misinformation. To address it, we built a fourth structural equation model that examined the theoretical linkages among government trust, misinformation exposure, misinformation elaboration, presumed influence of misinformation, and support for government restriction of misinformation.

As Figure 11.4 illustrates, misinformation exposure affected elaboration of misinformation, which led to presumed influence of misinformation, which in turn prompted respondents to support government restrictions of misinformation. In this particular model, government trust was treated as a moderator that affected the relationship between misinformation exposure and presumed influence of misinformation and the relationship between presumed influence of misinformation and support for government restriction of misinformation. That is, trust in government would enhance or attenuate the effect of misinformation exposure on presumed influence of misinformation. The higher or lower the level of trust in government, the stronger or weaker the relationship between misinformation exposure and presumed influence of misinformation. Similarly, trust in government would enhance or attenuate the effect of presumed influence of misinformation on support for government restrictions of misinformation. The higher or lower the level of trust in government, the stronger or weaker the relationship between misinformation exposure and support for government restrictions.

To test the model, we employed a structural equation model. Results of the SEM showed that the model fit was adequate ($\chi^2 = 513.80$, $df = 84$, $\chi^2/df = 6.17$, $p < .001$; CFI = .99, TLI = .98, NFI = .98, RMSEA = .035). The model explained 6.1% of the variance in exposure to misinformation, 26.5% in elaboration of misinformation, and 14.9% in support for government restrictions of misinformation. In terms of strengths of the linkages among the variables in the model, exposure to misinformation had a significant and direct impact on misinformation elaboration ($\beta = .25$, $p < .001$), presumed influence of misinformation ($\beta = .16$, $p < .001$). Misinformation elaboration had a significant and direct effect on presumed influence of misinformation ($\beta = .45$, $p < .001$), and support for government restrictions of misinformation ($\beta = .27$, $p < .001$). Finally, presumed influence of misinformation had a significant and positive effect on support for government restrictions ($\beta = .17$, $p < .001$).

The moderating role of government trust in the relationship between misinformation exposure and presumed influence of misinformation was tested using the PROCESS macro model 1 (Hayes, 2017). The results indicate that there was a significant interaction between misinformation exposure and government trust, indicating that the effect of misinformation exposure on

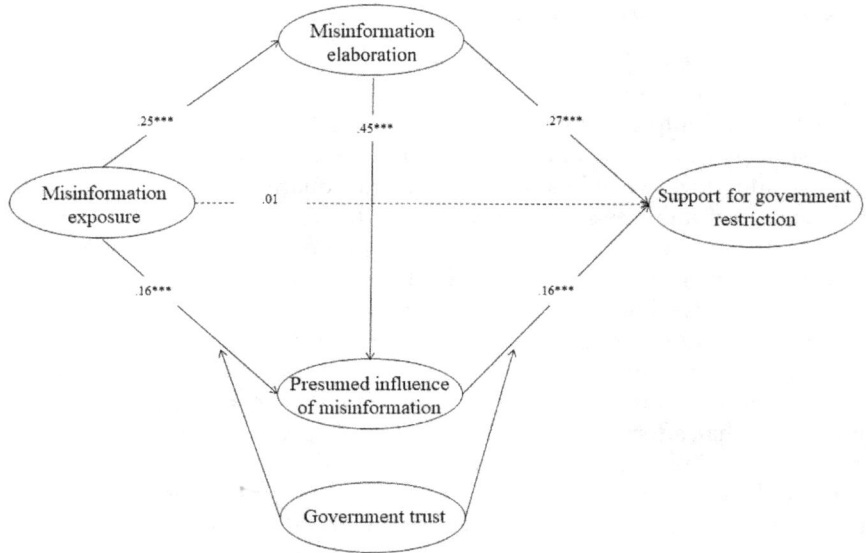

Figure 11.4 Structural equation model of predictors of support for government restrictions of misinformation with government trust as a moderator.

presumed influence of misinformation was moderated by government trust (β = .086, *SE* = .02, 95% CI = [.054, .117]). These results indicate that government trust enhanced the effect of misinformation exposure on presumed influence of misinformation. The relationship between misinformation exposure and presumed influence of misinformation became stronger as the level of government trust increased.

Following the same approach, the moderating role of government trust in the relationship between presumed influence of misinformation and support for government restrictions of misinformation was also tested using the PROCESS macro (model 1). It is interesting that results of the analysis indicate that government trust significantly but negatively moderated the relationship between presumed influence of misinformation and support for government restriction of misinformation (β = −.104, *SE* = .01, 95% CI = [−.129, −.070]). It means that trust in government diminished the effect of presumed influence of misinformation on support for government restrictions of misinformation. The relationship between presumed influence of misinformation on the public and support for government restriction of misinformation became weaker as the level of government trust increased. Conversely, the relationship between presumed influence of misinformation on the public and support for government restrictions of misinformation became stronger as the level of government trust decreased.

These results indicate that the effect of misinformation exposure on the presumed influence of misinformation varies by the level of government trust.

When the trust in government is high, a higher level of exposure leads to a greater level of projected harms of misinformation to the general public. The results are consistent with findings in Chapter 7—trust in government was a counterweighing factor, while exposure to misinformation was a contributor to the respondents' anti-vaccine attitudes. The results also underscore that the respondents' support for government action in restricting misinformation related to COVID-19 on social media was subject to how much trust they had in the government. The conclusion to be drawn from these results is that trust in government interacts with exposure to misinformation in jointly impacting the respondents' cognitive, attitudinal, and behavioral responses to the misinformation.

Summary of Key Findings

The key findings of the structural equal analyses are summarized. They reveal the dynamic process and effects of COVID-19 misinformation society with the underlying causal mechanisms of several mediators and moderators. Specifically,

- Information accessibility was a significant but negative predictor of exposure to COVID-19 misinformation and perceived interest of others. Moreover, exposure to COVID-19 misinformation and perceived interest of others were significant positive predictors of misinformation-sharing behaviors. These findings indicate that exposure to COVID-19 misinformation and perceived interest of others are significant mediators of the relationship between information accessibility and misinformation-sharing behaviors. It appears that increased exposure to COVID-19 misinformation and perceived interest of others caused by information accessibility led to more misinformation sharing.
- Information accessibility was significantly and negatively associated with exposure to COVID-19 misinformation and misinformation sharing. Exposure to COVID-19 misinformation and misinformation sharing were significant predictors of misinformation beliefs, anti-vaccine attitudes, and knowledge about COVID-19. That is, information accessibility was related indirectly to misinformation beliefs, anti-vaccine attitudes, and knowledge about COVID-19 through the two mediators—exposure to COVID-19 misinformation and misinformation sharing,
- To explore the presumed influence of COVID-19 misinformation on respondents' behavioral responses, our integrated model based on the influence of presumed influence model and the information-processing theory shows that information accessibility affected levels of exposure to misinformation, which led to elaboration of misinformation, which led to presumed influence of misinformation, which elicited negative emotions, which in turn prompted respondents to take restrictive, promotional and correction actions. Further, presumed influence of misinformation

on others was directly and indirectly related to support for government restrictions, promotional behavior, and civic actions to counter misinformation with negative emotions as the mediator. The greater the presumed influence of misinformation on others, the greater the negative emotions. The greater the negative emotions, the greater likelihood of support for government restrictions of misinformation, for sharing correct information about the pandemic, and for countering misinformation.
- Trust in government moderated the relationship between exposure to COVID-19 misinformation and presumed influence of misinformation on others. The relationship between exposure and presumed influence became stronger as the level of government trust increased. In addition, trust in government also moderated the relationship between presumed influence and support for government restrictions of misinformation. That is, the relationship between presumed influence and support for government restrictions became weaker as the level of government trust increased.

A Caveat in Order

Although the results concerning the theorized relationships we examined in this chapter were considered as causal, it does not necessarily mean certainty in causality in the four SEMs. To ascertain the cause-and-effect relationships, additional data, such as panel surveys, or different research methods, such as controlled experiments, are needed. Thus, the results of this chapter need to be interpreted with caution.

The cost of the COVID-19 global pandemic on economy, the general public's health and its well-being are enormous. In the next and final chapter (Chapter 12), we will summarize the significant findings from survey data and focus group discussions to draw conclusions. The practical implications, including the takeaways for public policymaking, will also be recapped for the benefit of fighting against misinformation in future public health crises.

References

Bagozzi, R. P., & Yi, Y. (2012). Specification, evaluation, and interpretation of structural equation models. *Journal of the Academy of Marketing Science, 40*(1), 8–34. https://doi.org/10.1007/s11747-011-0278-x
Bollen, K. A. (1989). *Structural equations with latent variables.* New York, NY: Wiley. https://doi.org/10.1002/9781118619179
Gunther, A. C., & Storey, J. D. (2003). The influence of presumed influence. *Journal of Communication, 53*(2), 199–215. https://doi.org/10.1111/j.1460-2466.2003.tb02586.x
Gunzler, D., Chen, T., Wu, P., & Zhang, H. (2013). Introduction to mediation analysis with structural equation modeling. *Shanghai Arch Psychiatry, 25*(6), 390–394.
Hayes, A. (2013). *Introduction to mediation, moderation, and conditional process analysis: A regression-based approach.* New York, NY: The Guilford Press. https://doi.org/10.1111/jedm.12050

Hayes, A. (2017). *Introduction to mediation, moderation, and conditional process analysis: A regression-based approach*. New York: Guilford Publications.

Kulesa, A., Krzywinski, M., Blainey, P., et al. (2015). Sampling distributions and the bootstrap. *Nature Methods, 12*(6), 477–478. https://doi.org/10.1038/nmeth.3414

McGuire, W. (1978). An information processing model of advertising effectiveness. In H. Davis & A. Silk (Eds.), *Behavioral and management science*. New York, NY: Ronald Press/Wiley.

Sobel, M. E. (1982). Asymptotic confidence intervals for indirect effects in structural equation models. *Sociological Methodology, 13*, 290–312. https://doi.org/10.2307/270723

12 An Asian Perspective on Combating Misinformation

What Have We Learned?

Ran Wei

What Have We Learned from the Study in Combating COVID-19 Infodemic?

The infodemic has hit Asia just like the rest of the world. We documented in this book the emergence and spread of misinformation during the COVID-19 global public health crisis. Because misinformation is characteristically short, catchy, and visually appealing, it has posed a huge challenge to public health officials in China (Beijing), Hong Kong, Singapore, and Taiwan (Taipei) in controlling the pandemic. Additionally, misinformation appears to come from nowhere with no URLs or sources to trace. The half-truths about COVID-19 spread cyclically, erupting in bursts and peaking repeatedly during the pandemic. We further found that misinformation makes people angry, worried, anxious, and annoyed. The more they encounter misinformation on social media, the stronger their negative emotions, which adds to the woes of the public's mental well-being.

From the stimulus-reasoning-orientation-response perspective (refer to Chapter 1 for the framework), we examined the process and effects of encountering misinformation. We focused particularly on the public harms attributed to the widely proliferated misinformation under different social-political systems and information environments, which condition the emergence and spread of misinformation. As a stimulus, misinformation causes people to engage in sense-making and prompts a range of responses (for an overview of our research design, refer to Figure 1.1 in Chapter 1). A striking pattern has emerged from the results of the cross-societal analyses presented in Chapters 4–10—the gap in the diffusion of misinformation and the uneven public harms of misinformation across the four studied cities.

First, a structural difference across the four cities is access to digital information on social media. Our studies indicate that as a macro-level structural factor, digital information accessibility plays a pivotal role in shaping the exposure and diffusion of COVID-19 misinformation in a society. That is, the greater access to digital information, the less exposure to misinformation during the first year of a global public health crisis. At the same time, the freer the information flow during the crisis, the less sharing of misinformation.

DOI: 10.4324/9781003355984-12

In China, which is characteristically media-rich and information-poor (Wei et al., 2018), restricted access to digital information on social media resulted in a scarcity condition, forcing respondents living in Beijing to view as much as information online as they could to stay informed, unfortunately including misleading, unverified, and factually incorrect information about the coronavirus. In this information-scarce environment, Beijing respondents shared the limited information with those around them, including misinformation, more often than did their counterparts in Hong Kong, Singapore, and Taipei. On the other hand, in societies with free access to rich and diverse information such as Hong Kong, Singapore, and Taiwan, citizens viewed less misinformation. We attribute the uneven pattern of diffusion to the free flow of digital information and the marketplace of ideas. Consistent with our past studies (Wei & Lo, 2021), these findings from the four societies with markedly different media environments underscore the role of digital information accessibility in shaping the public's encounters with misinformation.

Thus, a key lesson is that access and transparency are the necessary social conditions for understanding the diffusion and consequences of encountering COVID-19 misinformation on social media. A conclusion to be drawn from the varied diffusion pattern of misinformation is that unrestricted access to digital information is critical in combating infodemic during a public health crisis. Free and unrestricted access empowers citizens with timely and rich information they need to filter out half-truths and separate falsehoods from truth. Evidence from our cross-societal analyses suggests that limiting access to digital information is counterproductive.

A second lesson is that the public harms of encountering COVID-19 misinformation across different societies may be uneven. Across a range of outcomes, the negative effects of misinformation on respondents in Beijing, Hong Kong, Singapore, and Taipei appear to be *differential*, subject to the larger societal context—the greater the information accessibility, the less exposure and sharing as well as fewer negative cognitive and attitudinal effects. Conversely, restricted access leads to greater exposure and sharing, which contributes to negative emotions, anti-vaccine attitudes, misbeliefs about COVID-19, and knowing less about the pandemic.

To recapitulate our key findings from Chapters 6 to 10 on structural differences in access to misinformation: Beijing respondents who were the most exposed to COVID-19 misinformation among the four cities reported the highest level of overall negative emotions. Their mental well-being fell victim to the misinformation. The harms of misinformation on citizens' cognitive abilities in society appear to be similar. The negative effects of the misinformation in hindering the public's acquisition of factual knowledge about the pandemic are less in societies with free access. But in information-poor societies with restricted access, citizens cannot get sufficient information resources to cope with the public health crisis, and their cognitive capabilities tend to be harmed more (e.g., more likely to accept false claims as true).

It is worth noting that the gap in the diffusion is closely related to the pattern of uneven harm to the public. As our SEM analyses in Chapter 11 indicate, access to digital information and exposure to misinformation jointly affect citizens' emotions, risk perception, beliefs about misinformation, attitudes toward vaccination, and actions to counter misinformation. These results indicate that societal and structural differences prevail over individual-level factors in understanding the processes and effects of COVID-19 misinformation. We consistently found that Beijing respondents were exposed the most to misinformation and were the most impacted in terms of anxiety, anti-vaccine attitudes, and knowledge of the pandemic. Conversely, their counterparts in Taipei had the fewest encounters with misinformation and were least affected by the encounters.

Therefore, a third lesson is that free access not only empowers citizens with information but it is also beneficial to the public in mitigating the harms of misinformation in society. The more restrictions, the greater the public harms.

Fourth, the trust that citizens put into their public institutions plays a positive role in battling COVID-19 misinformation by counterweighing the harmful consequences of consuming and engaging with misinformation. For example, in Chapter 7, we found that trust in government diluted the public's anti-vaccine attitudes. That is, trust in government was a sort of counterweighing factor while exposure to misinformation was a contributor to the respondents' anti-vaccine attitudes. Considering that mass vaccination drives are essentially initiated by the government, confidence in the government can enhance the public's evaluation on the effectiveness of vaccines, thus boosting positive attitudes on vaccination. This particular revelation was an unexpected bonus of our research—trust in government helps fight the public harms of misinformation during a public health crisis.

Finally, average citizens are by no means totally powerless to deal with the tsunami of misinformation on popular social media platforms they visit. At the individual level, the harm is not even, either. The degree of harmful effects of misinformation varies, subject to user characteristics. Our findings consistently show that the more the respondents were knowledgeable about the coronavirus, the less they shared COVID-19 misinformation, and the less they accepted false claims made in the misinformation. Moreover, knowing something factually correct about the pandemic facilitated gaining more correct knowledge about it.

Additionally, encountering misinformation about COVID-19 may stimulate citizens' actions to contest misleading claims. Those thoughtful and better-educated respondents were particularly active in fighting misinformation. At the same time, respondents with a high-level knowledge fact-checked misinformation more often than did those with a low-level knowledge. Our cross-societal analyses showed that Beijing respondents who were exposed to misinformation and shared it with others the most frequently were the most active in fighting back. Thus, a fifth conclusion we have reached is to flatten the curve, knowledge is power—a well-educated and knowledgeable public is critical to this.

All things considered, the cross-societal findings suggest the following remarkable pattern, which highlights the trajectory of COVID-19 misinformation in four of Asia's leading societies: *Unequal access to digital information leads to uneven diffusion of misinformation, which results in different harms to the public.* We believe that findings of this cross-societal and interdisciplinary study deepen the understanding of a key societal factor—access to digital information—that accounts for the uneven level of exposure to and spread of COVID-19 misinformation and the differential impacts of the misinformation on citizens' risk perceptions, beliefs, attitudes, and knowledge in the four Asian societies.

In short, what we can learn from the cross-societal analyses is broader than pinpointing the specific public harms of misinformation; it is the confluence of macro socio-political-cultural factors and individual circumstances that need to be taken into full account.

Asian Perspective on Combating the Emergence and Spread of Misinformation

Our cross-societal analyses of COVID-19 misinformation in four major Asian cities provide an Asian perspective, which are characterized by: (1) an emphasis on hardware at the expense of social-techno software; (2) the government as a solution to the infodemic; and (3) government pandemic-control policy as a driver of the dynamic process and effects of misinformation.

1 The four societies studied represent a wide segment of Asia's political spectrum from authoritarian rule to viable Western-style democracies. In between, there are variations of authoritarianism with varying levels of political participation and civic freedoms. The control of misinformation showcases a government's—particularly an authoritarian government's—emphasis on developments of IT hardware (e.g., infrastructure, networks, and devices) at the expense of the software of social-techno conditions (e.g., marketplace of ideas, unrestricted access, and free flow of information). Asian countries are among the world's best equipped in terms of building modern IT infrastructure and networks. Hong Kong and Singapore are models of high-tech cities. The adoption rates of smartphones and smart devices in this part of Asia are among the world's top. However, with tight control of access to online channels and exchange of information on social media platforms, the social-techno conditions of using the IT technology fall short of the ideals of new media technologies serving as marketplaces of ideas and of equal access to information. When the infodemic hit Asia in 2020, the citizens living under restricted access encountered more misleading half-true messages than did those living with free access. This is an irony—in the most restricted societies that

limit the free flow of digital information, the spread of misinformation is greater, and the negative impact of misinformation on the public is the most unequivocal.

2 In the Asian cultural context, the general public's confidence in the government as a solution to infodemic exemplifies high institutional trust. With regard to the state-society relationship, the political culture in East and Southeast Asia is traditionally what Shi (2015, p. 9) called "hierarchical orientation to authority." According to the Edelman Trust Barometer (2022) reports, trust in the government and public institutions tends to be high in most Asian societies, with some exceptions such as Hong Kong where trust in government has become low in recent years due to the social and political turmoil that occurred prior to the outbreaks. In our findings, the role of institutional trust in reducing resistance to vaccination and support for government action to control COVID-19 misinformation is indicative of the Asian perspective in fighting infodemic. The extent to which the proliferated COVID-19 misinformation is harmful to citizens rests upon the level of public trust in government. Across the board, support for the government action to restrict misinformation by legislation was the most favored action among the 4,094 respondents. Thus, the expected government-as-solution is a unique aspect of combating misinformation in the four societies of our study.

3 Government pandemic-control policies drive the dynamic process and effects misinformation. After enduring the pandemic for almost three years, the general public has suffered fatigue. Thus, a government's approach to controlling the pandemic has far-reaching bearings on the citizens' mental well-being. When we connected the telephone survey data on exposure to COVID-19 misinformation with the different pandemic policies employed in the four cities (i.e., zero-COVID policy in Beijing vs. living with the virus strategy in Singapore vs. dynamic zero-Infection strategy in Hong Kong and Taipei), we found additional evidence of the negative impact of misinformation on citizens' well-being—exposure to misinformation was significantly related to the mental state of overload, which was the strongest predictor of information avoidance. That is, misinformation tends to worsen the overload problem. It also indirectly motivates citizens to avoid information altogether.

On the other hand, the dynamics driving the process and effects of misinformation changed. The web survey data revealed that respondents in Singapore under the living with COVID policy were the most exposed to information about COVID-19. Not surprisingly, they were the most overloaded. Respondents in Beijing living under the strictest zero-COVID policy encountered less of such information; and their information load was lighter than their counterparts in Singapore. Pakhomov (2022, p. 1) argued that the political cultures of East Asian countries exemplify the highest form of the state's "total power." Our findings in this large-scale study underscore the role of government policy in driving the dynamics process and effects of misinformation in the late stage of the pandemic.

In conclusion, revealing an Asian perspective on combating infodemic with the above characteristics is not only a unique advantage of our studies but it also reflects the socio-political-cultural landscape in the four Asian societies.

Recommended Actions for Public Policy

Informed by the key findings and insights from the conclusions, we end this concluding chapter with a set of recommendations for coherent public policy to combat misinformation in future public health crises:

At the infrastructure level, the Asian perspective suggests that updates in IT hardware needs to go with improvements in software. For example, improving the social-techno conditions by establishing a marketplace of ideas, platforms of information exchange, forums of public information resources, and providing free access to digital information—all of these IT soft-side capabilities are critical in effectively controlling the diffusion of misinformation. Freely accessible information will arm citizens with timely, rich, and diverse information to cope with a public health crisis and make them less vulnerable to harms from misinformation. Setting up firewalls to block and restrict access to digital information will be counter-productive.

In building these informational forums and exchange platforms, transparency is the key. As we have shown in big data analytics, it is very difficult to eliminate misinformation because it comes from nowhere and spreads fast on decentralized social media sites. Transparency with information during a crisis, however, will shrink the space for rumors, fake news, and misinformation to gain footing. In addition, transparent and timely information enables the public to filter out falsehood from truth or fact check misleading claims. The benefit of online information will be less when accessibility is restricted and timely and rich information is in short supply. Thus, we recommend that public health authorities and medical experts maintain open and transparent communication with the public, especially on digital media platforms. As soon as misinformation appears on social media platforms, factual and evidence-based information should be presented promptly so that the general public can fact check user-generated content to sort out inaccurate or false information.

Establishing space for public deliberation, Q&A, and debate is equally important to access. Public health authorities should plan campaigns with a focus on delivering provocative messages that facilitate the public's deep thinking or elaborative processing. When people can deliberate over and discuss misinformation, negative cognitive effects can be attenuated. By Q&A and debating, citizens can gain accurate knowledge to build their necessary literacy to cope with the crisis. As we found, better-educated citizens who take efforts to process the misinformation they encounter on social media are most active in fighting back.

Further, sources for timely and accurate information about a public health crisis need to be clearly identified as official. Trust in public institutions enhances people's acceptance of updated and factual information from public sources. For instance, timely communications and guidelines from the government can increase people's willingness to get vaccinated. Timely and accurate information presented by authoritative sources, such as health agencies, should reduce the encounter of misinformation that might gain popularity via sharing.

At the individual level, a well-educated public is critical to flattening the curve of the infodemic. Education can be a powerful tool in preparing and equipping the public with the ability to form accurate perceptions about the public health risks. For instance, citizens with a high-level knowledge about the pandemic tend to do more fact-checking of misinformation than do those with a low-level knowledge. Thus, it is important to educate the general public with infodemic literacy campaigns that improve public knowledge supported by scientific or fact-checked information. In addition to the civic infodemic literacy campaign, public health authorities and government agencies should correct misinformation as soon as it is spotted. An effective and sustainable way to combat misinformation during a public health crisis is to improve citizens' resilience to misinformation through timely debunking or correction practices and proper literacy education programs.

Finally, we note the importance of mobilizing citizens to take civic actions in combating misinformation. Our findings suggest that citizens' action is particularly critical to overcome the waves of false, misleading, and factually incorrect information on popular social media platforms. In particular, the government and public health officials should energize better-educated citizens to contest misinformation. To assist the citizens, public health websites and social media posts need to provide detailed factual information to arm citizens with the needed knowledge to identify and debunk half-truths during a pandemic.

A Word of Caution

Governments need to walk a fine line: Although being informed about pandemic situations with sufficient updated and scientific information is crucial for pandemic control, public health officials need to pay attention to the phenomenon of "too much" information, especially among older people and males. Too much information may cause overload, and information overload causes citizens' intention to avoid information. Thus, more information can be counter-productive.

To keep the public informed, public institutions involved in the prevention and control of pandemics need to consider setting a limit on the amount of information they send out for public consumption. Also, public health agencies need to monitor updates and daily briefings to avoid a breaking point of providing too much information.

References

Edelman Trust Barometer. (2022). *Trust in China*. Retrieved November 10, 2022, from https://www.edelman.com/trust/2022-trust-barometer/trust-china

Pakhomov, O. (2022). *The political culture of East Asia: A civilization of total power.* Singapore: Springer. https://doi.org/10.1007/978-981-19-0778-4

Shi, T. (2015). *The cultural logic of politics in mainland China and Taiwan*. New York, NY: Cambridge University Press. https://doi.org/10.1017/CBO9780511996474

Wei, R., Huang, J., & Zheng, P. (2018). Use of mobile social apps for public communication in China: Gratifications as antecedents of posting articles on WeChat public accounts. *Mobile Media & Communication, 6*(1), 108–126. https://doi.org/10.1177/2050157917728100

Wei, R., & Lo. V. (2021). *News in their pockets: A cross-city comparative study of mobile news consumption in Asia*. New York, NY: Oxford University Press. https://doi.org/10.1093/oso/9780197523728.001.0001

Appendices
Appendix 1.A

List of text mined debunked misinformation messages about COVID-19 in four cities

Misinformation narrative	SM platforms	Cities
1 Mosquitoes can transmit the COVID-19 virus.	Weibo/Facebook/Twitter	Beijing/Hong Kong/Taipei
2 5G mobile networks can transmit the COVID-19 virus.	Weibo/Facebook/Twitter	Beijing/Hong Kong/ Taipei/Singapore
3 Drinking alcohol can kill the COVID-19 virus.	Weibo/Twitter	Beijing/Taipei
4 Non-inactivated COVID-19 vaccines will alter human DNA.	Weibo/Facebook/Twitter	Beijing/Hong Kong/ Taipei/Singapore
5 Asians are more prone to COVID-19 infection than others.	Weibo/Twitter	Beijing/Taipei
6 Omicron cannot be detected by PCR test.	Weibo/Facebook/Twitter	Beijing/Taipei
7 Many countries announced the cancellation of all quarantine procedures, COVID-19 tests, compulsory vaccination and are henceforth considering COVID-19 as flu.	Weibo/Facebook/Twitter	Beijing/Hong Kong/Taipei
8 Masks can be reused after boiling or alcohol disinfection.	Weibo/Facebook/Twitter	Beijing/Hong Kong/Taipei
9 Drinking a large amount of water and keeping one's throat moist can help prevent infection.	Weibo/Facebook/Twitter	Beijing/Hong Kong/ Taipei/Singapore

(Continued)

(*Continued*)

Misinformation narrative	SM platforms	Cities
10 Garlic and ginger can help improve immunity and prevent infection.	Weibo/Facebook/Twitter	Beijing/Hong Kong/ Taipei/Singapore
11 Saline gargling can prevent infection.	Weibo/Facebook/Twitter	Beijing/Hong Kong/Taipei
12 Taking hot showers can prevent infection.	Weibo/Facebook/Twitter	Beijing/Hong Kong/Taipei
13 Shower head can transmit coronavirus.	Weibo/Facebook/Twitter	Beijing/Hong Kong/Taipei
14 Prolonged use of N95 masks can cause oxygen loss of 5–20% and may lead to hypercapnia.	Weibo/Twitter	Beijing/Taipei
15 Maintaining the body in weak alkalinity can fight COVID-19.	Weibo/Twitter	Beijing/Hong Kong/Taipei
16 People who are vaccinated are more likely to be infected by Omicron.	Weibo/Facebook/Twitter	Beijing/Taipei
17 Vaccinated individuals shed new COVID-19 strains.	Weibo/Facebook/Twitter	Beijing/Taipei/Singapore

Appendix 1.B

Sample profile of web surveys in the four cities (N = 4,094)

Key demographics	Beijing (n = 1,033)	Hong Kong (n = 1,017)	Taipei (n = 1,019)	Singapore (n = 1,025)
Age (in years) (mean, SD)	39.90 (11.80)	39.48 (12.84)	39.36 (13.08)	42.70 (14.46)
Gender (male) in %	49.30	45.10	47.70	51.10
Education attainment in %				
High school or lower	12.70	25.90	13.70	20.20
Vocational school	22.70	14.40	16	23.80
Bachelor's degree	59.40	51.60	53.50	45.90
Master's degree or higher	5.20	8.10	16.80	10.10
Income (in USD) in %				
$0–1,566 (Beijing) $0–2,564 (Hong Kong) $0–1,079 (Taipei) $0–2,189 (Singapore)	8.10	10.80	8.10	13.80
$1,567–3,133 (Beijing) $2,565–5,128 (Hong Kong) $1,080–1,797 (Taipei) $2,190–5,109 (Singapore)	27.80	26.90	14.90	30.20
$3,134–4,700 (Beijing) $5,129–7,692 (Hong Kong) $1,798–2,516 (Taipei) $5,110–8,029 (Singapore)	25.30	26.90	15	26.40
$4,701–6,266 (Beijing) $7,693–10,257 (Hong Kong) $2,517–3,235 (Taipei) $8,030–10,949 (Singapore)	19.40	20.70	16	15.60
$6,267–7,833 (Beijing) $10,258–12,821 (Hong Kong) $3,236–3,954 (Taipei) $10,950–13,869 (Singapore)	13.70	8.40	22	7.90
$7,834 or above (Beijing) $12,822 or above (Hong Kong) $3,955 or above (Taipei) $13,870 or above (Singapore)	5.70	6.40	24	6.10

Appendix 1.C

Sample profile of telephone surveys in the four cities (N = 4,114)

Factors	Beijing (n = 1,000) M (SD) or %	Hong Kong (n = 1,008) M (SD) or %	Taipei (n = 1,056) M (SD) or %	Singapore (n = 1,050) M (SD) or %
Age, years (N = 4,076) (mean, SD)	44.79 (14.27)	48.67 (16.37)	53.58 (16.34)	41.15 (13.96)
Gender (male) in % (N = 4,114)	54.30	50.20	42.70	48.60
Education in % (N = 4,092)				
High school or lower	27.90	51.20	27.10	25.50
Vocational school or non-degree program	22.80	9.70	16.30	31.70
Bachelor's degree	39.10	29.20	40.10	35.30
Master's degree or higher	10.20	9.90	16.50	7.50

Appendix 1.D

Framework for developing focus group protocols

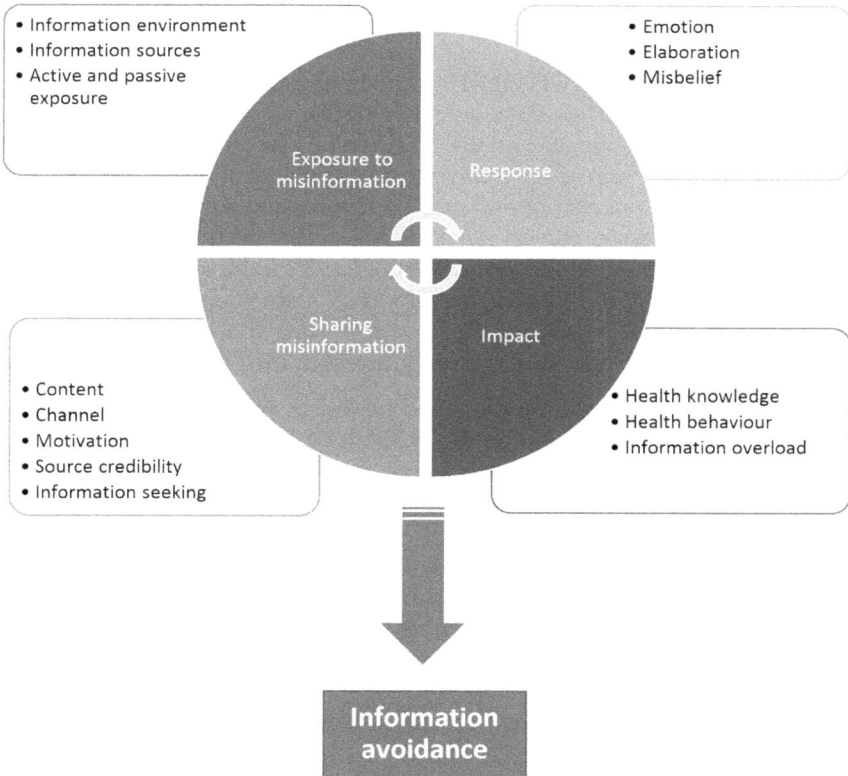

- Information environment
- Information sources
- Active and passive exposure

- Emotion
- Elaboration
- Misbelief

Exposure to misinformation

Response

Sharing misinformation

Impact

- Content
- Channel
- Motivation
- Source credibility
- Information seeking

- Health knowledge
- Health behaviour
- Information overload

Information avoidance

Appendix 1.E

Structured moderator guide for focus groups

1 Exposure to misinformation

1 (Priming)

- Think about all COVID-19-related information that you obtained during the last few days, weeks, months, or years. What is the most "ridiculous" one to you? By "ridiculous", we mean, this information sounds very untrue but many people just believe in it; OR this information sounds very true but later on it turns out to be untrue; OR this information sounds very shocking but you don't know whether it is true or not, even not until today. (Reminder: It can be something related to COVID vaccine, control measures, any news you read from the mass media or social network, facts (or non-facts) about COVID-19, etc.)
- Please share with us and write it down in the "chat box" (in zoom)

   NOTE: Everything discussed below, as written in "this informa-tion" should be based on the "COVID-19-related information" that they share in the "chat box" here.

2 Information environment/information sources

- Where did you get **this information** (information sources, for instance, mass media, social media, and personal networks)?
- Who was/were the source(s) of such information? Government or health agencies, health professionals, opinion leaders, friends, and family?
- Why do you think it is "ridiculous"? (Explain, and need to provide contexts)

3 Active or passive exposure

- How did you get **this information**? Were you intentionally seeking for it from XXX (e.g., the news media? Social network? Family? Friends? Or else?)

   Probes:

- If the participant sought for the information "intentionally" (or actively), please ask why did s/he do so? Did s/he often try to find information related to COVID? If yes, why? If no, why did s/he seek this particular information actively?
- If the participant did not seek for this information; meaning that s/he received the information passively. Ask her/him, how did s/he feel when heard about/received this information? Did they feel "lucky" or "annoyed" by hearing about COVID? If yes, why?
- How often did your family or friends try to share COVID-related information with you? Do you think they shared too much/ too little information with you? Why? (Note: Here, the COVID-related information can be anything related to COVID.)

4 Misinformation

- How do you know whether this information is true or false? What did you do to check the accuracy or authenticity of the information?

Probes

- If someone mentions, "fake news," or "misinformation," or "rumor," etc., please ask: How do you know this is a XXX? Could you please recall any other misinformation, rumors or fake news you have heard of?
- If no one mentions these, please ask them: Have you ever heard of the term, "misinformation" (or "infodemic"? or "disinformation", "mal-information")?
  - If yes, please ask them to define: What is "misinformation"? How do you define misinformation? Could you recall any misinformation you encountered during COVID-19?
  - If no, ask them about the "rumors" or "fake news" they have heard of about COVID-19. Could you please recall any of the rumors or fake news you have heard of?

2 Responses

1 Emotions

- How did you feel after you heard of this information (negative emotions such as sad, worried, fearful, angry, anxious, etc., OR positive feelings such as relieved, safe, relaxed, etc.)?
- Why did you feel that way (Please ask the participants to explain why they had such feelings)?

2 Elaboration

- What did you think of this information when you read it? How did you decide if the information is accurate (or false)? Did you do any fact check? Or google? Or ask around?

3 **Misbelief**

- Have you ever believed in some COVID-19-related information/news, while later found out that they are not true or even fake?
- If yes, how did you find out? What did you do to deal with it?

4 **Information seeking and sources credibility**

- What information sources/channels do you rely on when seeking COVID-19-related information?

  Probe:

- If the participant says they searched for information, ask:

  - Is there any particular source of information you trust? Why?
  - Is there any particular source of information you do not trust? Why?

- If the participant didn't search for information, but, for example, just naturally "knew" or "heard about" COVID-19-related information, ask:
  - Which sources do you rely on to get COVID-19-related information? Why do you pick up this source(s) to track the current pandemic situation?

  - For participants who rely upon social media or social network sources, ask them how often they use social media/social network to obtain information, how much attention they pay to these media/social network, and how often people from their social network/social media share information via such platforms? What do they usually share? Is there any discussion or confrontation they can recall?

- Is this source(s) reliable? Why do you think it is/isn't?

  - if someone preferred to receive information from a source s/he didn't think reliable, ask them (1) why they are still using this source and (2) if there is any source they consider reliable
  - if someone thinks a source is a reliable one but not using it, ask why

3 **Impacts**

1 **COVID-19-related knowledge/health information**
2 **Health behavior (vaccination)**

- Whether you are vaccinated or not, have you ever searched for information related to the COVID-19 vaccines?
- Have you had any concerns over getting a vaccination?
  Probe

  - If yes, what are the concerns? How did they affect your decision on getting a vaccination?

- If no, how did you convince yourself to be or not to be vaccinated? What did you do to convince yourself?
- (For all participants) Did you search for any information related to these particular concerns?
- If yes, ask: What did you do to search for the information (for example, google, seeking advice from professionals they know, checking information from health authorities)?
- If no, ask: Why not? How did you ultimately deal with the concern?

3 **Information overload and avoidance**

- Do you still search for COVID-19-related information recently?
- Do you think there are too much, too little, or just about right amount of COVID-19-related information out there?
  - If answer "Too much," ask why? Could you please describe

4 **Sharing**

1 **Objectives**

- Have you ever shared the information you mentioned? Whom did you share with? Through what channels? Why did you want to share it with them?
- Do you usually share COVID-19-related information? Could you give us one example? Who do you share with? How often do you share?

2 **Motivation**

- Why do you want to share/not share COVID-19-related information?
- Are there any concerns about sharing COVID-19-related information?

3 **Response**

- How did they react/respond when you shared that information? Were they interested? Was there any discussion or confrontation?
- What did you think of these reactions/responses?

4 Perception of health policy
  1 How would you describe COVID-19-related health policy in your society? "Zero COVID"/ no-tolerance COVID policy or coexisting with Coronavirus?
  2 What do you think about these different styles of health policies? Which do you prefer? Why? Where did you get the information you mentioned?
  3 Do you discuss COVID-19-related policy with others? Did you share the information you mentioned with them? How did they react/respond when you shared that information? Is there any discussion or confrontation?

Appendix 2.A

List of keywords pertaining to COVID-19 misinformation posts on Weibo

Keywords in English	Keywords in Chinese
rumors \ rumor \ misinformation \ believing rumors \ false \ fake news \ false information \ conspiracy \ pseudoscience \ title party \ fabricated information \ unsubstantiated information \ misleading information \ factual error \ diffuse truth \ no research evidence \ no groundless accusation \ nothing factual basis \ disregard of facts \ open mouth \ solemn statement \ confuse right with wrong \ almost believed \ do not confuse	谣言\传言\流言\错误信息\谣传\误传\信谣\传谣\造谣\辟谣\不要相信\假的\不实\假消息\虚假信息\阴谋\伪科学\标题党\失实信息\捏造\未经证实\误导性信息\事实性错误\扩散真相\传闻\无任何研究证明\无端指责\毫无事实依据\罔顾事实\信口开河\严正声明\混淆是非\差点信了\切莫混淆

Appendix 2.B

List of extracted topics and representative keywords from Weibo by frames

Topic	Sub-topic assigned by LDA	n (%)	Keywords	Translation
COVID-19 origin	9, 14, 16, 17, 21, 25	56,650 (19.81%)	病毒, 武汉, 新冠, 病人, 零号, 研究所, 黄燕玲, 回应, 发布, 感染, 信息, 声明, 肺炎, 近期, 冠状病毒, 新型, 工作, 网络, 毕业生, 流传, 新冠, 病毒, 感染, 确诊, 报道, 病例, 研究, 发现, 患者, 时间, 疫情, 肺炎, 研究所	Virus, Wuhan, New Crown, Patient, Zero, Research Institute, Huang Yanling, Respond, Post, Infection, Information, Statement, Pneumonia, Recent, Coronavirus, Novel, Work, Network, Graduate, Spread, New Crown, Virus, Infection, confirmed, reported, cases, research, found, patient, time, outbreak, pneumonia, institute
Virus infection cases	22, 28	16,501 (5.77%)	感染, 男子, 小区, 人员, 出门, 接触, 买菜, 医生, 武汉, 确诊, 肺炎, 医院, 发现, 患者, 网传, 发布, 病例, 检测, 核酸, 阳性, 确诊, 感染, 患者, 病例, 患者, 病毒, 疾控, 中心, 北京, 冠状病毒, 新型, 病例	Infection, Man, Community, Personnel, Going Out, Contact, Grocery Shopping, Doctor, Wuhan, Diagnosed, Pneumonia, Hospital, Found, Patient, Internet Transmission, Posted, Case, Detected, Nucleic Acid, Positive, Confirmed, Infected, Patient, Case, patient, virus, CDC, center, Beijing, coronavirus, novel, cases

(Continued)

(*Continued*)

Topic	Sub-topic assigned by LDA	*n* (%)	Keywords	Translation
Pandemic updates	6, 29	14,059 (4.92%)	病例, 确诊, 新增, 密切接触, 治疗, 累计, 隔离, 肺炎, 报告, 疑似病例, 出院, 死亡, 接受, 医学观察, 治愈, 输入, 新型, 检测, 病例, 防控, 确诊, 新闻, 发布会, 记者, 数据, 工作, 情况, 武汉, 湖北, 患者	Cases, Confirmed, New, Close Contact, Treatment, Cumulative, Isolation, Pneumonia, Report, Suspected, Discharged, Death, Accepted, Medical Observation, Cure, Imported, Novel, Detection, Case, Prevention, Confirmed, News, Released meeting, reporter, data, work, situation, Wuhan, Hubei, patients
Virus spreading	5, 10	15,635 (5.47%)	疫情, 新冠, 病毒, 快递, 千万则, 杀灭, 流传, 春节, 开放, 停运, 茶水, 病毒, 新冠, 疫情, 传播, 新型, 冠状病毒, 肺炎, 感染, 防控, 宠物, 人类, 证据, 传染, 在家	Epidemic, New Crown, Virus, Express, Never, Kill, Spread, Spring Festival, Open, Out of Service, Tea, Virus, New Crown, Epidemic, Spread, New Type, Coronavirus, Pneumonia, Infection, Prevention and Control, Pet, Human, evidence, infection, at home
COVID-19 information publicity	0, 2, 8, 23	43,575 (15.24%)	北京, 检测, 消息, 人员, 疫情, 发布, 信息, 官方, 记者, 工作人员, 上海, 医院, 证明, 相关, 流传, 防疫, 疫情, 肺炎, 新冠, 发布, 汇总, 警方, 信息, 传播, 依法, 发布, 人员, 通报	Beijing, Detection, News, Personnel, Epidemic, Release, Information, Official, Reporter, Staff, Shanghai, Hospital, Prove, Relevant, Spread, Epidemic Prevention, Epidemic, Pneumonia, New Crown, Release, Summarize, Police, Information, Spread, According to Law, publish, personnel, inform

(*Continued*)

(*Continued*)

Topic	Sub-topic assigned by LDA	*n* (%)	Keywords	Translation
Pandemic prevention	3, 4, 20, 24, 27	43,260 (15.13%)	新冠, 病毒, 预防, 新型, 冠状病毒, 口罩, 病毒感染, 疫苗, 防护, 感染, 熏醋, 疾病, 预防, 抑制, 茶叶, 免疫, 人体, 呼吸道, 建议, 接触, 症状, 自来水, 加大, 静置, 注入, 氯气, 口罩, 病毒, 酒精, 防护, 喷洒, 飞沫, 水分, 颗粒, 分离出来	new crown, virus, prevention, novel, coronavirus, face mask, virus infection, vaccine, protection, infection, vinegar smoked, disease, prevention, suppression, tea, immunity, human body, respiratory tract, advice, contact, symptoms, tap, increase, stand, inject, chlorine, mask, virus, alcohol, protection, spray, droplets, moisture, particles, isolate
Virus detection	18	10,660 (3.73%)	核酸, 憋气, 肺部, 30秒, 检测, 患者, 医院, 肺炎, 出院, 阴性, 治疗, 新型, 冠状病毒, 确诊, 感染, 医护人员, 标准, 武汉, 症状, 两次	nucleic acid, hold your breath, lungs, 30 seconds, detection, patient, hospital, pneumonia, discharge, negative, treatment, novel, coronavirus, confirmed, infection, medical staff, standard, Wuhan, symptoms, twice
Policies and measurements	1, 26	19,281 (6.73%)	工作, 防控, 疫情, 做好, 措施, 管理, 期间, 人员, 保障, 时间, 服务, 相关, 组织, 确保, 安排, 通知, 防控, 疫情, 人员, 口罩, 检测, 核酸, 病例, 新冠, 做好, 防护, 健康, 工作, 风险, 肺炎, 隔离, 聚集, 佩戴, 社区	work, prevention and control, epidemic situation, do a good job, measures, management, period, personnel, safeguard, time, service, related, organization, ensure, arrange, notify, prevention and control, epidemic situation, personnel, masks, detection, nucleic acid, cases, new crown, do well, protect, health, work, risk, pneumonia, quarantine, gather, wear, community

(*Continued*)

(*Continued*)

Topic	Sub-topic assigned by LDA	n (%)	Keywords	Translation
Political issue	13	16,715 (5.85%)	特朗普, 疫情, 确诊, 夫妇, 新冠, 希望, 真的, 感觉, 医生, 隔离, 首相, 柬埔寨, 中国, 洪森	Trump, Epidemic, Confirmed, Couple, Corona, Hope, Really, Feeling, Doctor, Quarantine, Prime Minister, Cambodia, China, Hun Sen
Social impact of pandemic	12	5,284 (1.85%)	市场, 板块, 指数, 辉瑞, 涨幅, 今日, 疫苗, 经济, 上涨, 震荡, 资金, 跌幅, 点击, 概念, 美股, 风险, 股票, 科技, 全球	Market, Sector, Index, Pfizer, Gains, Today, Vaccines, Economy, Rise, Concussion, Funding, Decline, Clicks, Concepts, US Stocks, Risk, Stocks, Technology, Global
Vaccination	15	18,173 (6.35%)	疫苗, 辉瑞, 新冠, 美国, 临床试验, 接种, 公司, 瑞德, 西韦, 试验, 治疗, 研究, 报道, 药物, 临床, 副作用, 公布, 批准, 数据, 研发	vaccine, Pfizer, COVID, USA, clinical trial, vaccination, company, Reid, civir, trial, treatment, research, report, drug, clinical, side effect, announcement, approval, data, research, and development
International aid	11	14,496 (5.07%)	蒙古国, 捐赠, 中国, 湖北, 人民, 疫情, 启动, 新闻, 隔离, 二连浩特, 首批, 检疫, 蒙古, 中方, 羊肉, 入境, 屠宰, 羊, 抗击, 上海	Mongolia, Donation, China, Hubei, People, Epidemic, Startup, News, Quarantine, Erenhot, First Batch, Quarantine, Mongolia, China, Lamb, Entry, Slaughter, Sheep, Fight, Shanghai
Others	7, 19	11,673 (4.08%)		

Index

Note: **Bold** page numbers refer to tables; *italic* page numbers refer to figures.

For Product Safety Concerns and Information please contact our EU
representative GPSR@taylorandfrancis.com
Taylor & Francis Verlag GmbH, Kaufingerstraße 24, 80331 München, Germany

* 9 7 8 1 0 3 2 4 1 0 4 7 0 *